I0704400

CONTRACEPTION ABORTED

Life Begins At Contraception

Luke John

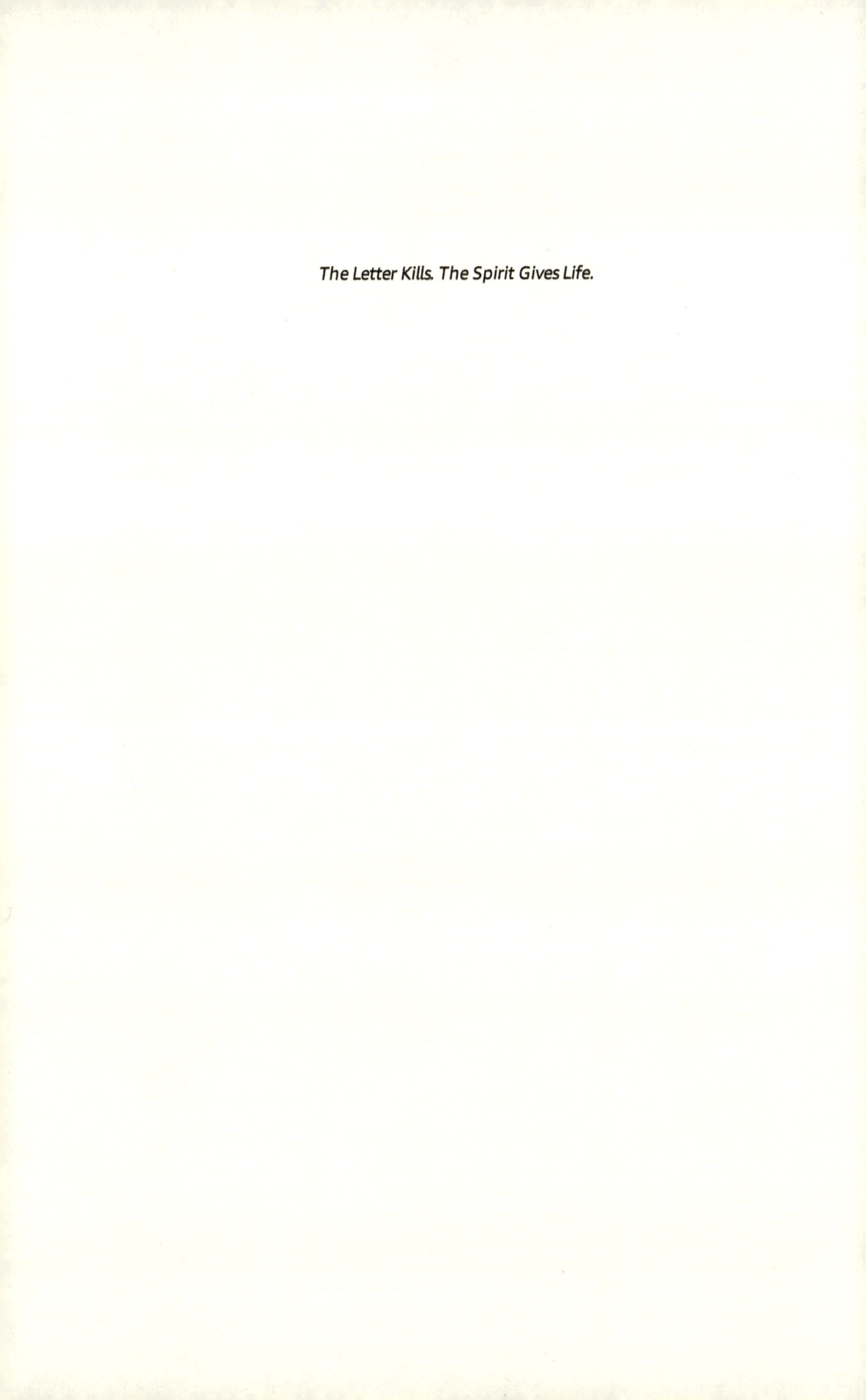
The Letter Kills. The Spirit Gives Life.

Copyright © 2020 Luke John

All rights reserved.

Children are first conceived in the mind.

CONTENTS

PREFACE

Children are first conceived in the mind. Their motto is "Life begins at contraception." Our abortion debate centers on children and their quality of life. For the decades since Roe v. Wade, the pro-life, pro-choice wall has committed us to ideological, trench warfare. This book tries to peek around that wall, by making the fetus a little more mature than normal. The fetus adds a personal voice for consideration. Think of a young child privy to and intimate with adult quarrels. Although the unborn know about civil rights, they discuss abortion mainly in the context of adult responsibility. They believe life begins at contraception. They explore the links between themselves and pre and postnatal health services. They focus on the quality of their intended childhood. The unborn, somewhat selfishly, came up with their very own lobby called pro-baby. They have their peculiar list of demands for the adult population. These include unborn social security. They assume all newborn life is a deliberate decision, not coital collateral damage. In this book, the unborn know the abortions continue to happen. They know the abortion issue is perennial. They see a need for emotional closure. There is, however, this formidable wall of divide. They go around the wall. We follow them.

THE ABORTION OF CONTRACEPTION.

The leader of a major world power, while at an undisclosed country resort, goes jogging. He manages this without a security detail. His attire, sweat vests, short pants, jogging shoes, a camouflage cap, and a nice wristwatch. Half an hour into his jog, a man emerges from the cover of some bushes and assaults him. DNA later confirms a gentleman arrested as the attacker.

Primetime that very night. Many talk show hosts, replace the staple fare of paranormal, asexual, meteorite fortified, vega-carne-trophic moms, with the comparatively normal subject of an assaulted president. The president's folly in being out alone, in the quiet countryside, is much decried. "The president is an idiot." One host educates. "He deserved it," the audience roars back. Wild applause erupts, without even a cue from the applause lights.

In his office one week later. The president, still unable to sit comfortably, stands. His clothes are immaculate, but his mind is a state of disarray. Yes, maybe he brought all of this upon himself. "God!" He asks himself, "Why?" He struggles to ignore the explanation noised by some political colleagues. How could they? Why would they? How dare they suggest he harbored a subconscious, secret desire to have a homosexual encounter?

For the first time, he understood the military's old, "Don't ask, don't tell" policy. He didn't want anyone, including his wife, to ask about the incident. Like hell, he didn't want anyone to tell. This he realized was a vain hope. His abuser had already secured an advance, and a book contract to tell all.

Hell, he thinks, why not just declare himself a federal disaster area? He needs all the help in the world now, but so little is forthcoming. His party thinks of him as a political liability. Fraud accusations, the political machinery can deal with that. It's merely water under the bridge. Sexual harassment charges yes, a president can survive that, and come out happily on top. An abused president? Hmm. It was this very morning that the vice president had hinted at her willingness to, "Restore the American image to its former dignity." She was speaking of their imminent policy reassessment on climate change and free trade. Make America exceedingly great again, she had concluded. Nothing changed how deflated and slumped he felt. Like a used crumpled bathroom napkin. He felt he was waste. Toxic waste.

He reasoned he had brought all of this on himself. Alone, flimsy clothes, the funny smiley face watch, and male. He had asked for it. That was for sure. The Secret Service special agent. Man, was she easy to remember. "Don't you read the news? What on earth possessed you to allow this to happen? Alone? If you were not still the president..." She composed herself. "Sir, I would chew you up for being an idiot." He readily agrees. He does not qualify to expect help. The painful puffiness of his right eye is comfortable, compared to the brittle anguish dwelling in his stitched right cheek.

One thing pleases him. He is no longer in hospital care. Those chiding, accusing glances. The solitude of his office suited him just fine. Let them snigger. Let them laugh. In here, he would never overhear their coarse wit. Better yet, his open eye would never see the condemnation plastered onto every face.

The coffee was cold now. There was no need to touch or taste it. He just knew. "Hell!" His tortured mind echoed. "Hell!" The

President of the United States just does not get raped. That was the truth. There was no need to reason this out. He just knew it to be so.

Pain wracked mind and body. He almost did not have to feel it, he just knew. The press dogs were busy. The editors were even busier. The reports had to be just right. The president had to know they supported him. He deserved to understand that all America suffered with him. The wording had to be just right. Yes, a sexually handled president sold advertising space. The editors knew that. The literary agents and writers knew that. The readers knew that. "Aw, he should have been more careful."

The president slides a stack of briefings, on abortion and contraception, to the side. This would be for yet another tomorrow. He reaches in a desperate appeal to touch his beloved American flag. His bruised fingers clutch at the fabric. This was America. He would find justice here. Old Glory, that Star-Spangled Banner, would never betray a compromised, worsted, and broken citizen. He remembers its hope and strident faith in the triumph.

"And why that Star-Spangled Banner flies.
The sacred shed substance of patriots.
The honored, and the unknown who died the sacrifice.
Bloodied toil sweated into national prosperity.
Acres of ideals cultivated into world envied freedom.
That's what we are. And what are we?
The flag and the pole. That's what we are.
The flag pole to that living banner."

Was he still a part of that living banner? He did not feel a part. Not in the very least. He hopes, but not with much conviction. He crumples an end of the flag into his fists.

"A fabric woven for healing."

The president stands still, time stands at attention. He does not feel like a pole anymore. The flag needs a more worthy bearer. The flag deserved better, and it was not for his slow response to employment and health issues. There was no one to turn to. Thank God. He had the quiet of his office, and the flag to cry on. But this time, even the flag would not heal.

Time reverses. Again, the rude rag barricades his mouth and nostrils. He loses consciousness, but only just. His captor wants him awake, but not very much so. Again, fists cuff at him. Again, his face inhabits dirt and turf. Repeatedly, a heavy hand lowers onto his head. The flavor, of pain and blood, again decorates the taste buds of his brain. Again, he kicks and struggles. The uncouth hand of oppression grinds his face into the dirt. Moments later, handcuffs click. He is a prisoner to that wayward mind. Again, his shorts rip. Again he dies.

Now, through the haze of stinging tears and shameful memories, the president resolves to reclaim honor. His shame-surfeited mind decides dignity or death. The president knows he is being unreasonable, in blaming himself for raping himself. Terror strikes with an unmerciful impact. He considers the social reaction. His status has plummeted, he is no longer president. He is only a rape victim.

What differentiates rape from ordinary assault, he questions? People suffer abuse daily. He knew. He read the crime briefings. There was the sex factor, but that was not it. His regard, for his society, ripped his face into untidy shreds of guilt and fear. The society was not tolerant of, nor sympathetic to sexually manhandled individuals. The president, as president knew that. As a professional crowd-pleaser, the president feels unable to resist the conventional wisdom. Not even to preserve his sanity. He makes peace not with himself, but with his society. He agrees the rapist has destroyed his life and sexuality. He agrees and dies some more.

Even while the president's tears bathe the flag, America continues with sociological and psychological analysis. The young man is a victim of emotional deprivation. A feminist mother mangled his adolescence, pundits conclude. The poor child fulfilled her subliminal command, "Desecrate the alpha male." The poor kid. Why did the president have to make it so easy for him? Poor boy, why did the president have to hurt him so?

Still in the Oval Office, the president stares fixedly into the gray nothingness of his numbed mind. He moves his face to a bullet defying window. His raspy exhalations assault the pane. What is there to see? He knows not. Still, he stares. Outside, a sunlit world glares. Then he sees it. A difficult smile creeps onto his cheeks. He surveys the security of his office. "No," he again concludes, "The President of the United States does not get raped."

LIFE BEGINS AT CONTRACEPTION.

They had both enjoyed the hours of the foreplay. The unfettered exploration of merged passions. Together, they had coyly coaxed each other. They had strolled, hands entwined, to the mountains of orgasmic delights. It was a few months later, at another time. The growing baby was theirs, and the pregnancy was all hers.

This is another story, about another time and another place. It was Texas 1969, when (Jane Roe) considered a then legal impossibility. Abortion. A woman's life had to be at stake, for the longhorns of Texas law, to permit an abortion. Life at stake did not then extend to modern frivolities, like current emotional, or future psychological distress. You needed to be in mortal danger, in the most normal interpretation of the word. Burnt at the stake, at stake. If the issue were not abortion, one could well quip, "We've come a long way, baby." After Roe v. Wade, it seemed so simple, so settled, so clear. We know, from the many abortion protests and legislative battles, it is not so simple, so settled, or so clear. Even as the world grapples with the pandemic Covid-19, no abortion ceasefire is as yet declared. Humanity is global, reproduction is universal, and children are everywhere. It is reasonable to suppose people, outside of Texas, also think about and discuss abortion.

In full Hazmat gear, let's go up to Canada, cool off, and prepare for a world tour. We will experience various abortion laws and reproductive health realities on our trip. Every nation has its abortion story. Let's start somewhere random. Say the Isle of Man, which swims in the Irish Sea. The first leg of our tour is short. El Salvador, Columbia, Argentina, Brazil, Nigeria, Zaire, South Africa, Sudan, Ethiopia, The Russian Federation, India, China, Norway, Italy, France, Germany, Singapore, The Philippines, Indonesia, Australia, New Zealand, Barbados, Jamaica, and the Commonwealth of Dominica. We drop by the Middle East, and do a full tour there, then let's stop in Mexico. From the Estados Unidos Mexicanos, let's consider again what's going on with abortion, just north of the border. After a USA stopover, we shall continue our meticulously planned global tour.

Back to 1973. The United States Supreme Court gave birth to Roe v. Wade. Roe v. Wade established abortion rights, even in abortion tough states like Texas, Iowa, Louisiana, and Tennessee. The US Supreme Court made the right to a first-trimester abortion a constitutionally protected, private medical transact. A woman, according to Roe v. Wade, no longer needed to be near death's gurney to have an abortion.

This is from the 1973 Roe v. Wade decision: section X1. Source. FindLaw.

"To summarize and to repeat:

1. A state criminal abortion statute of the current Texas type, that excepts from criminality only a life-saving procedure on behalf of the mother, without regard to pregnancy stage and without recognition of the other interests involved, is violative of the Due Process Clause of the Fourteenth Amendment.

(a) For the stage prior to approximately the end of the first trimester, the abortion decision and its effectuation must be left to the medical judgment of the pregnant woman's attending physician.

(b) For the stage subsequent to approximately the end of the first trimester, the State, in promoting its interest in the health of the mother, may, if it chooses, regulate the abortion procedure in ways that are reasonably related to maternal health.

(c) For the stage subsequent to viability, the State in promoting its interest in the potentiality of human life may, if it chooses, regulate, and even proscribe, abortion except where it is necessary, in appropriate medical judgment, for the preservation of the life or health of the mother.

2. The State may define the term "physician," as it has been employed in the preceding paragraphs of this Part XI of this opinion, to mean only a physician currently licensed by the State, and may proscribe any abortion by a person who is not a physician as so defined.

In Doe v. Bolton, post, p. 179, procedural requirements contained in one of the modern abortion statutes are considered. That opinion and this one, of course, are to be read together.

This holding, we feel, is consistent with the relative weights of the respective interests involved, with the lessons and examples of medical and legal history, with the lenity of the common law, and with the demands of the profound problems of the present day. The decision leaves the State free to place increasing restrictions on abortion as the period of pregnancy lengthens, so long as those restrictions are tailored to the recognized state interests. The decision vindicates the right of the physician to administer medical treatment according to his professional judgment up to the points where important state interests provide compelling justifications for intervention. Up to those points, the abortion decision in all its aspects is inherently, and primarily, a medical decision, and basic responsibility for it must rest with the physician. If an individual practitioner abuses the privilege of exercising proper medical judgment, the usual remedies, judicial and intra-professional, are available."

The feeling one gets from Jane Roe's application for access to legal abortion is simple. Ms. Jane did not want to kill anybody. At that point in her life, Jane just did not want to become a mommy again. Perhaps sometimes, when you're 21 years old and not feeling very settled, another baby just seems overwhelming. For the record, Ms. Jane gave birth to her baby before the Supreme Court ruled. Ms. Norma McCovey also died very much pro-life, according to the much-published record. From the grave, however, Ms. McCovey seems to have left us a documentary note that her pro-life volte-face was, in fact, a paid advertisement. The irony of it all would be whimsical. This is abortion. Nothing is whimsical about abortion. Roe v. Wade did not invent abortion or the debate. Roe v. Wade gave a legal choice to keep or not to keep. Roe v. Wade has no clause commanding women to have abortions. The logic is simple, for those opposing abortion. Abortion is wrong. The Court cannot make it right. We believe it is wrong and unlawful to abuse a child. We do not make exceptions for abuse within the privacy of the home, or the womb.

Let us start another conversation about the same abortion debate. There is one word frequently lacking. What lacks and ails in this perennial debate is the little word, Parent. Parent is no common noun. We debate life, law, morality, murder, holocaust, responsibility, and irresponsibility, God, Satan, good, evil, sin, just pure evil, and eternal life. What about Parents? Wars have proven the army won't miraculously lead itself. Let's make a few inquiries. Ask Mahatma Ghandi, ask Hannibal, ask Sun Tzu, and Martin Luther King. Ask Yamamoto, ask Taharqa, ask Rommel, ask Boudica, ask Chaka, ask Churchill, ask Patton, ask the historians. Ask Irene Morgan v. Commonwealth of Virginia, Ask Saladin, ask Genghis, ask Caesar, ask Sitting Bull, ask Carib Warner & Chatoyer, ask Alexander, ask Napoleon, ask Zhukov, ask Balla & Nanny of the Maroons, ask Fidel, ask L'Ouverture, ask Mussolini, ask Minor v. Happersett, ask Mandela, ask Washington, ask history itself. Compared to armies, with minimal adult input, children seem miraculously to survive.

Children like, armies and social movements, need a little help growing up. If the baby survives boot camp, we finally end up with an adult. This brings us back to the P-word. Parent. We could make it simple. "No law shall compel another person to become a parent. Anyone who wishes not to be a parent shall not be hindered in such pursuit." We could assume this fallacy rather safely. Children would prefer if their parents (plural) greatly, actually, happily, wanted and desired them. Anything else seems sort of routine, multicellular propagation. Could precious, sacred children be collateral coital damage?

We are all here, however temporarily, because we were born. We can have opinions because we were born. Critically, we have survived long enough to consider events and issues, even those like abortion. If the pro-choice were never born or had all died in infancy, we'd have no abortion debate. Children would still need responsible, stable parents. Those conceived would conceivably appreciate a secure and functional upbringing. Children may even venture to desire a little love and affection, as a special topping, while growing up. An end to abortion does not supply children with willing or responsible parents. Is it the right inviolate of the State to impose, compel, or otherwise demand parenthood? Is it our social jurisdiction to demand others become parents?

Conception might be a mostly cerebral event. When our parents (plural) want us, we are conceived. The assumption is they want us for our benefit and for a good cause. When sperm fertilizes an egg, we unequivocally have biological fusion. Conception is quite another event. Pregnancy is the process that gives birth to the conception. Is our vaunted appreciation of human life to equal the fusion of pre-programmed, viable DNA? We can perform this life miracle in a petri dish, or a teacup. We are not speaking of the possibility of human cloning, like that famous Dolly sheep. Nature has conception down to a science. Fertilization is usually a very predictable event in the fallopian tube.

Without our very "consent" we get pregnant. Once the ingredients meet, nature manages our fertilization affairs. All life forms reproduce somehow. We may have sufficiently evolved beyond reproduction. There is the small matter of nurturing our reproductive prospects. As we affirmed earlier, children need parents, not just successful gestation & birth. It is the manifest destiny of children to have parents. It is optional to become a parent. Christians have Jesus to reference. It's routine to legislate the legality, or illegality of abortion. It has proven a little more difficult to legislate the love, care, and time children need, once they are born. What is a child's recommended daily allowance for love? Do they even need this social vitamin, anyway? Do children get malnutrition of the soul, if poorly cared for?

Religious people know how difficult it is to find a little love in this world. The case law on the reality of human civilization is overwhelmingly available. In both secular and religious flavors, youth are an endangered species. As for our enlightening world tour. We did not get to speak with as many officials as we hoped. My fault. We, however, got to meet very many children and parents. They were literally everywhere. So, who cares about all these silly little children? Parents do. I am wrong. Sometimes, parents don't about their children.   Sometimes parents can't care for their children. Children, always need care.

THE JOB IS FAMILY.

Contraception Aborted defines conception as the moment, adults decide, it is an intelligent time for expanding family. Bill of Right: No right exists to impose parenthood on the unborn child. Parenting is an all-volunteer mission. No conscription, no forced labor. Somewhere in antiquity, the abortion moment conceived and continued to reproduce. The Abortion World War is from unborn generation to generation. Pro-life versus pro-choice is kin to the trench warfare of World War One. Ideologically the lines got drawn, the boundaries set, and the legal attrition exercised daily. Both the giving of birth, and having an abortion speculate, in unborn futures. Abortion unambiguously ends the future. Our future is the hope of a stable, happy family. Well, let's be realistic. A child can't exactly hope for the luxury of happiness. An education and enough to eat should suffice. After all, we grew up on so much less. See us now. We did fine for ourselves.

According to a Wikipedia article, The Apocalypse of Peter, extant August 2016. We see the fate of women who have abortions detailed. "Women who have abortions are set in a lake formed from the blood and gore from all the other punishments, up to their necks." This fate is just like normal life, for some women. They expose the woman's head, so the, understandably peeved spirits, of the unborn, can shoot flashes of laser-guided fire into the eyes of these women. This is the hell destined for women who indulge in abortions. No press release yet, if repentance changes the woman's fate. Some claim the writing is from the second century A.D. So even from ancient times, abortion and the corresponding judgment is intimately, if not exclusively, a female hazard.

The Guinness Book of World Records may accept former real estate mogul, Donald J. Trump, as the most inconceivable politician since Empress Catherine the Great of Russia. Mr. Trump's inauguration as the 45th, President of the United States of America was January 20th, 2017. Before Donald Trump was Roe v. Wade. In his bluntly spoken straight talk, he made it all simple. He would strategically shuffle the United States Supreme Court's deck of Justices. A conservative (pro-life inclined) majority of Supreme Court Justices would overturn Roe v. Wade. He may not be right, but he was clear. Build the Abortion wall. Perhaps the children will pay.

Let us go a wee bit back in time. Before Barak H Obama became the first. Before America made itself great again. Before the coronavirus pandemic. There was September 11th. This event weighed in on matters other than suicide bombers and terrorism. Leaders of industry hung up on corporate calls and hustled home to handle family business. Mothers became moms and called up long-estranged teenage offspring. Love ridiculed the stoic code of manly conduct. Dads kissed, hugged, and cried comfort to equally emotional sons. The word dysfunctional was temporarily dropped from family. As if by executive order, the love flowed. The World Trade Center towers crumbled and smoldered into remarkable, monumental ruin. America unabashedly loved and prayed.

In 2016, the United States Supreme Court's, 5 to 3 decision in Whole Woman's Health V. Hellerstedt, struck down the Texas House Bill of 2013. The HB2 abortion restriction laws imposed new regulations for the operation of abortion facilities. The stated intention of the proposed law was to protect women's medical welfare. It required abortionists to have admitting privileges at a nearby hospital, and for clinics to have improved surgical facilities. What in the whole wide world can be wrong with improving the healthcare provided to women? What can be wrong with protecting unborn children from pain? It is important to research the motive of our legal transactions. We get to see intent. We would not let our love manifest itself, with undue burden, procedure, ritual, and convolutions designed only to frustrate. The nonexistent Jesus Christ complained about privileged persons imposing heavy legal burdens. We can read his imaginary biographers Mathew et al. The abortion battle rages on.

It is May 2020 and the US Supreme Court is doing the legal magic on June Medical Services v. Russo. This suit seeks an overturn of a Louisiana law. The Louisiana Unsafe Abortion Protection Act ("Act 620.") As if legal déjà vu, the Louisiana act requires abortionists to maintain active admitting privileges with a hospital within thirty miles from where they operate. Roe v. Wade expects state law not to impose any undue burden on women seeking abortions. Motivation for these new regulations stem, it is said, from one Dr. Kermit Gosnell. A jury of his peers convicted American physician Kermit Gosnell in May 2013 of murdering three infants who were born alive, and of involuntary manslaughter of a lady who died because of an abortion procedure. Mr. Gosnell according to the evidence ran a practice "Women's Medical Society," injurious to the public, predatory, and disreputably, and incorrigibly self-serving. Still, for all his failings, his crime was not abortion and the killing of unborn children. He just killed badly.

You wonder what happens when a baby is born. Must children be born with a thirty-mile radius of a hospital? Must all midwives have admitting privileges? Because of early childbirth. Should mothers find residence in an area no further than thirty miles from a hospital? This would only be for five weeks before their due date? Sometimes a law is too inconvenient to be worth the law. Legislatures are there to make laws. It is their right. Nobody will die because of Prohibition, or bans on contraception, or the advertising of the same. It changes how we live.

Abortion is ultimately about how unborn children will live. If peradventure they are born. Our laws should do more than manage us. Good laws are indiscriminate with benefits. And yes the Supreme Court stuck 5 to 4 with its precedent and overturned the Louisiana law. What bothers, is the energy we invest in ensuring children are born to unwilling parents.

Towards the end of the 18th century or thereabout, the British Industrial Revolution gave birth to the modern era. Underground coal mines gave steam to another world of machinery. Mines picked apart by the innocence of British youth supplied essential fuel to the spirit of innovation and of invention. It was there, while swimming in sewers of surplus, humanity cautiously crept in. The adult conscience reluctantly massaged itself, to regard and protect the earth's little urchins. On 4th, August 1842, the British Parliament passed the Coal Mines Regulation Act, to end the use of children younger than ten in underground mines. Social progress is profound, spectacular, sweeping, and generous in its improvements. Let the record show. Society improves the lives of its children by dramatic leaps and bounds. Not these little baby steps, with which we have improved weapons technology. As recently as the American Civil war a 12 pounder cannon was considered a devastating, and game-changing implement of war. That we now have intercontinental ballistic missiles is just another normal fact of our times. The lives of our children has changed too. They can now drink lots of formula and look at TV from their cribs.

In 1933 or hereabout, Adolf Hitler dreamed of a German living space filled with healthy, genetically sound, German children. A noble wish, undoubtedly. No more of Mien Kampf (My Struggle) for the itsy bitsy babies. National Socialism would solve all these structural burps and bumps. Hitler forced on man another New World. A master race and a resultant arms race. Adolf Hitler's legacy excited in 20th-century man distinct and near-universal disapproval for overt, systemic, state-sanctioned, eugenics, and mass murder. After the agony of World War II, humanity was born again. We were reborn, averse to the overt display of death and destruction. The Hiroshima syndrome. We can destroy, marginalize, and oppress each other, but discreetly.

Time marches on. Humans were being newly born into September and the year 2001, the 11th day. For one brief, yet eternal moment in time, the job was family. For a brief, yet an eternal moment, basic values of kinship, blood & family replaced the debonair materialism that is America. "Remember Pearl Harbor," was a rallying call, to avenge shed blood, and balm national pride. A primordial howling echoing the rage, the tumult, and abandon of battle, vengeance, retribution, and death.

September 11th induced a labor of love which produced a partial-birth, soon stillborn, of spiritual aspirations. In that moment of indiscriminate slaughter there conceived, in the instant, a somber appreciation for life, and the Spiritual Spark. Throughout the world, especially in the US, the focus was on family. Magnificent monuments to human prowess, the Trade Towers. So quickly had they descended into inelegant tangles of mangled debris and heaped up dust. What hope was there for the individual human standing, rather shakily, on twin pillars of brittle bone? The chastened among us found refuge in the intangibles of love and heavenly priorities. We found solace investing in the common stock and bonds of family and human relationships.

It was September 11th, 2001. In the United States, from sea to shining sea, tears flowed with the ease Niagara falls. Throughout America the job was family. On that day of dying and death, one issue disappeared momentarily into the closet of irrelevance. The issue was abortion. The United States and the civilized world with it stood staunchly in pro-life solidarity. We accepted then that building family required living beings. Television images showed falling, adult bodies grasping uncaring air for futile life. Those of us, further removed from death, held our breaths in desperate hope. So many adult lives aborted. So many dreams aborted. Too many families interrupted. On September 11th there was no room in the civilized for more terror, there was no room in the world for death, there was no room in the world for more hate, there was no room in the world for evil, and there was no room for another abortion. On September 11th there was room only for love and for family, and there was also some room for Jesus.

LIFE V. ROE
AND WADE

Now, the following rambling is mostly a true story. I was told it was. A friend asked a friend, "Is abortion right or is abortion wrong?" The young and animated couple debated, "Is abortion murder?" So, the two walked the dust along a two-lane highway and nagged away at their brains. With relentless, unyielding replays they questioned, "Is abortion murder? Is abortion murder? Is abortion murder? Is abortion murder?" The staccato of trapped echoes threatened to puncture the skull from inside out. The jabs of right and wrong battered with equal ferocity. Steps slowed from stride, to slack shuffle, to a standstill. For several minutes there was standing. Moving, only to shift featherweight from one leg to the next. Was abortion right or wrong? What was the answer? What was the complication? Are answers not supposed to be simple things? One thing was as clear as a brilliant sun. Just one thing. The abortion decision had to be right. Who cares if the law permitted abortion, or restricted it? As many employees, slaves, and political prisoners have discovered, the law is not always on your side. Finding the right decision, the proper conclusion, was the simple aim. This was the basic consideration. Is abortion murder? That was the question before the family court. Is abortion murder? Such hopelessness and helplessness.

A drowning person knows the urgent need to escape the watery grave. They will be equally conscious of how powerless they are to save themselves. Abortion, as a legal issue, seemed not in the domain of the individual citizen. It was more than a question. It was a peril. Some nations made abortion legal, others made it a heinous crime. A potential minefield where limbs of morality would vanish with a simple misstep. It was mandatory to find the right way. The walk had to be on a safe path. Future moral mobility demanded it.

They heaved in a few deep breaths. One did not exhale. One swallowed quiet contemplations. They exited the courtroom and the demands for a straight answer. They suspended their self-inflicted cross-examination, the affliction of self-flagellation & inquisition. That little quiet moment, with its muted breathing, numbed the mind into a sedate realization. They turned squarely to face each other, friend to friend. "You know what," one asked? "We are asking the wrong question."

"True," the other rejoined, "Are you ready to be a parent?" We have had human behavior legislated for so long, we sometimes forget to think for ourselves. Whatever we think, we must understand this simple truth. People can get beheaded, arrested, excommunicated, and ostracized, for their contrary, naughty thoughts and deeds. Do, garden variety, bad parents exist? Do terrible parents exist? Why are immoral people allowed to have our innocent, vulnerable children? Do we have the time to raise other people's children? Do children get ill-treated, sometimes, at the designated institutions and places of safety? Is childbirth always the responsible decision for those dedicated, loving, married parents? Is it love to heap a burden of sinful conscience on them for using contraception? Are we sowing the seeds of depression and self-destruction, by condemning that congenital defect abortion? Must Christian women feel less committed to their Savior since that abortion?

Let us suppose 2019 AD recorded the last act of domestic abuse. It occurred in international waters at midnight on December 25th, 2019. This United Nations initiative was, with alacrity, ably supported by the World Conference of Churches, the Arab League, the Organization of African Unity, The Association of Southeast Asian Nations, the Organization of American States, The European Union, Britain, The Commonwealth, the Asia Cooperation Dialogue, CARICOM, NATO, the Warsaw Pact among others. 2019, the year eternal for joyous memories. 2019, the blessed year, the United Nations declared the world child neglect and abuse-free.

There is our sociology to add to abortion, as much as there is medical science. All humans share a similar mechanism for pregnancy and childbirth. Fetal viability is a medical and legal cornerstone. Hypocrisy is our sociological cornerstone. We know by now, the purpose of pregnancy is not to count uninterrupted trimesters. Hypocrisy translates well and with consistency, into any language, or creed, or culture. Hypocrisy requires no complex or expensive equipment to detect. We need a consistent, non-biased, guidance system to fetch a morally eloquent abortion answer. We must add up, not only multiply.

Abortion is a perpetual debate. Like a quarrelsome sibling, spouse, or neighbor. We have societies, frowning on a woman publicly breastfeeding a hungry baby.Breastfeeding is a private issue. Mothers must exercise discretion and social distancing. Mothers must plan for the inevitable hunger of their babies. Only rubber nipples allowed in public. We should wonder and aloud. How did abortion become a matter in the public domain? Even when we are unaware of a woman's pregnancy, motherhood is a communal affair. Why is abortion not a private matter handled discreetly? Shameful, when mere babes find themselves denied a wholesome milkshake. We have milk police because we pretend discomfort with monster breasts. We might want to re-examine the truth of our commitment to babies, and to life. Pilate may have famously asked Jesus, "What is truth?" Well, we at least know the truth does not lie.

THE PROCESS OF LAW. THE PROCESS OF PREGNANCY.

The due process amounts to oppression if the law itself is flawed. This could theoretically become law. Statute P 2: a measure to conserve scarce water resources. Be it known. Liquid bodily waste is now nationally approved as a breakfast beverage. A one to four ratio must be adhered to. Let us toast to the infinite legal possibilities. Let us pretend abortion is a jury trial. We could misdirect the jury, even though both sides have dutifully presented arguments for and against. We could say abortion is murder. We can also say based on our religious or cultural persuasions that abortion is always wrong, and never right. All we require from the jury is what punishments they think necessary for the crime. What does poor abortion have to say for itself? How does a reasonable society compel an individual to become a parent? There are times we expel pregnant girls from future formal education. Perhaps a little education might be a bit useful when raising children. We know the fact. Children need nurture, not just feeding. They have survived with chronic shortages of both. The unborn make no legal complaints, usually. The unborn present no mission statements. They, at our behest, embark on a lifelong mission called life. Who holds the first, the fundamental and inherent jurisdiction for unborn affairs? There is always the joy or the crisis of conception to contend with. Someone has to care for the child.

It was 1776. A political embryo, now a world superpower forced delivery on a rather mundane issue, "No taxation without representation". You can still hear all these grown men enraged. Their lives, livelihoods, and aspiration dictated without their input or consent. Before 1776 was 1773. Then the Massachusetts Sons of Liberty decided not to denounce the British Tea Act of May 10th, 1773 by walking up and down the muddy streets. They could have marched in peaceful protest with banners and placards. These practical folks had a Boston Tea Party, which involved boarding private property (ships) and destroying the cargo. Tea. Ah, why cry and fight over spilled tea?

We must understand. The American colonists were loyal British folks squatting overseas on Native American administered and occupied lands. These British citizens felt sufficiently empowered, by that natural gravitation to personal liberty, to agitate against the Crown. They rejected what they saw as intolerable and coercive legislation. British Parliament had passed laws following the Boston Tea raid, called the Coercive Laws, to bring the recalcitrant Englishmen in America to heel. By 1775 one of these laws, The Quartering Act of 1774, made provision for the housing of British soldiers in private dwellings. So much for an Englishman's house is his castle. The American colonist felt they were being strangled by the British crown. In their own words. "Prudence, indeed, will dictate that Governments long established should not be changed for light and transient causes; and accordingly all experience hath shewn, that mankind are more disposed to suffer, while evils are sufferable, than to right themselves by abolishing the forms to which we accustom them. But when a long train of abuses and usurpations, pursuing invariably the same Object evinces a design to reduce them under absolute Despotism, it is their right, it is their duty, to throw off such Government, and to provide new Guards for their future security." Source National Archives and Records Administration.

In our discussions on abortion. This I note. Abortion is no light and transient cause. We need to redefine abortion as a moral issue, and as a legal matter. The response of the British people living in America, to The Punitive Acts, was the American War of Independence. We could promote the view that the American War of Independence was illegal and immoral. It resulted, without doubt, in the death of viable living beings. This matter of life is an ideological war still being fought today. It seems natural for a nation conceived, begotten, and weaned on the concept of freedom, to safeguard personal freedom, personal destiny, and individual choice. In matters of parenthood, it seems civilized. There should be some tacit disconnect between our bodies and the State.

The State can make this abortion matter very simple. The State should not only ban abortion. The State should be proactive. It must regulate and legislate reproduction itself. Banning abortion truly multiplies the babies, but it does nothing to raise the quality, ability, capacity, willingness, or preparedness of the parents.

Start first, by telling citizens when to conceive. Just like with a draft. We'd register for national reproductive services but at puberty. It would serve the interest of the unborn and females that the State sanctions all new conception. Pregnancy, without an approved State permit or license, is illegal. It goes without saying. Only married persons qualify for permits, and only after rigorous psychological and financial analysis. We are very busy with abortion and murder. It seems we don't pay enough attention to the insignificant matter of parental duty. When a soldier can't perform his duty, we give him a discharge.

Children are a hopelessly dependent part of the social nucleus. As recently as the foundations of Rome. The head of the family, the paterfamilias, understood the fragility associated with having another mouth to feed, among other practical concerns. Exposure to the elements, aided by the ambiguous hands of fate, decided if the newborn lived or died. Now we are supercivilized. We preempt exposure mainly with contraception. Children can and have been born into a literal physical hell. They drown and they are burnt. We are not referring to the practice of child sacrifice, so vividly mentioned in the Holy Bible. Give the child a head start. Let the child start with willing parents. Children rely on their parents for things material, and things of emotional design. We might not want to compel a person to become or stay pregnant. Giving birth makes one a parent, in the most limited context of its definitions. We mislead ourselves, it seems, by equating reproduction to parenthood.

Contraception Aborted won't seek to address all abortion legislation and idiosyncrasies. Clarity exists in facts of basic medicine and sociology. We can only abort what is alive. Think of fire. One match is fire, it is not yet a campfire. A campfire is not yet an Australian Outback conflagration. Extinguishing the embryonic possibility of a wildfire seems prudent. Yes, a child is not a match. It appears a highhanded disservice, to the unborn, to compel their births. Our good intentions can never usurp the reality of our uncertain future. Our beliefs will not change the fact.

This is an evil world. The police and the judiciary think so. Life goes on until it ends. Giving birth is an open-ended, educated guess. We make this guess on behalf of our child guests. We of ourselves can do no better. The concept of family is a universal reality, whatever the local and cultural configurations. Abortion closes all possibilities. Birth provides access to many possibilities indeed. When we think it's worth the risks we become parents. It is yet hard to grasp this perverse worship of conception. It is no divine miracle for human beings, or goats, or rabbits to conceive. Pregnancy is a dangerous, yet routine and mundane business. Parenting requires classes.

The multiplicity of religious and intellectual persuasions proves we are in entrenched disagreement, as regards God. Here lies our freedom of conscience. We can hotly pursue our perdition, communally, or individually. Our salvation is our blessing. My choice directs me to the hell lane, your choice directs you to the paradise beachfront. My choice does not prevent you from winning the ultimate, holiness lottery. You have pleased your God. To reduce social discord, let the bodies of legislative influence reestablish the religious courts. We can say with misguided, yet with spiritually affected authority, "It is the will of God". Are we not infants struggling in our mission to curb child abuse? Are we not delinquent juveniles? To date, we remain hamstrung in our cause to dismantle the many cases of abuse against our beloved children. Our bid has failed to put a lid on the more obvious failings of child hunger and malnutrition. Lost in the daylight are we, managing the world's children.

Conception is a premise. Conception is an intellectual precondition for pregnancy. Similarly, there are conceptual drawings of projects and structural plans for our many projects. There is always the inevitable arrangement for project financing. All this work we do before the literal construction begins. We seem to reverse the process with children. Have the baby, then we'll figure things out. It is more like things will work themselves out. In the very best of times, the physical conception of newborn life is very much a calculated risk. Birth is a new and perilous journey for defenseless youth. No amount of rules and regulations will immunize a child from the effects of reluctant parenting. Suppose there was a child care deposit required to give birth. Many a woman would have to remain pregnant for years, as they scraped together the requisite birth price. Babies will push their way out of the womb, be it headfirst or breeched, heedless of mommy's finances. "Ready or not, here I come." Marriages delay, because couples don't feel financially stable just yet. What does it take to get married? Hopefully, consent and "I do," and two helpful witnesses.

Biologically conception grows, even when we are unaware of it. Conception's growth continues to the destinies of miscarriage or birth. Conception is not a spontaneity of nature, like a menstrual cycle. It takes a little inseminated effort on someone's part. There is no biologically mandated baby season. It should be a woman's right when to choose a pregnancy. This is an affirmative action. It should be a woman's right not to conceive. It is rather convincingly said, "It is her body." Well, is it? Women's fundamental right is to evade, delay, postpone, or renounce pregnancy if they so desire. We shall assume no one forces sexual intercourse and pregnancy on women. Life begins at contraception. However, our current abortion debate is about women claiming a right to become un-pregnant. Our authority to regulate and manipulate our reproduction derives from our sovereign authority over our person.

Pregnancy is not a spontaneous biological inevitability, like sundown and moonrise. We don't expect the womb to bring forth in its precise season a new baby girl or boy. Conception remains a personal, albeit collective biological construct. From even before conception, folic acid and issues of very unstable sociology loom relevant. The baby has an entire life ahead. The babies base their hopes on us. They hope we are well prepared. As the Apostle James says, "You know not what a day shall bring forth." Life lives, life dies. Both remain appropriately natural. Each within its context. Death's sneer terrifies perhaps most. Legends of reincarnation, of resurrection, of redirection, and immortality, and non-existence abound. The worst part about being born is not being able to pay the fee for the afterlife. Being born comes with lifelong personal responsibilities.

The concept of abortion is intuitively in disharmony, with our desire for life. No life means no possibilities. Logically so. It still puzzles. Why do folks, who assess others as unfit parents, want such people to procreate? Yes, we can force sterilization on them, but we won't allow abortions. Poor children. This takes us to the State mandated first degree, for having two to three children. A masters' degree for four or more, a diploma for one child only. In the event of twins, the diploma is acceptable with additional counseling. A Ph.D. for having no children.

Mankind has always had to manipulate nature and adapt to it. Reproduction is no sacred exception. Nature provides the air, the breathing is our choice. Nature presents the essential liquid. To drink filtered water is our decision. Hunger is of nature. Mealtime and nutrition is our choosing. The womb is natural. Conception is natural. Birth is natural. Parenthood is naturally our decision to make. Like conception, parenthood is not automatic. Both, while natural events, require definite contrived input to occur.

Let us drop anchor softly. Let us show we can calm, even a little, the perpetual waves which dash. Unattended our children surf the life. We agitate over the aborted unborn. They are bludgeoned by the horrors of circumstance. They are tortured by the sadism of deliberate neglect. The young continue to breathe in fear, grief, and trepidation. We are not discussing poverty here. Just parenting. It seems like the more chaotic, haphazard, and unplanned, a conception, the holier it is. The sanctity of life, much-touted, demands careful and reverent handling.

The manipulation of nature is an unavoidable responsibility. We have to interfere with nature. If we don't, we can forget earthquake and hurricane resistant buildings. Okay, we can go ahead and eat all our food raw, walk naked, sleep in caves, and in the open. Start fires from lighting or volcanic eruptions. Let the body eliminate its waste, on a need-to basis, whenever nature calls. Submission to the natural state is patently the natural thing to do. Especially embrace our natural state of nudity. Naked our mom delivered us. Death is conspicuously naturel. Yes, we were naturally born hungry. Feeding is another equation. Breast milk is consciously and purposefully fed to the baby. There is absolutely nothing automatic about becoming pregnant, or about caring for a baby. We are custodians of our reproductive time and seasons. Choose choices. We can choose wisely and with compassion.

Ring the bells, raise the polite voice, write the succinct legal brief, and resist inducing forced parenthood. Birth is a promise fulfilled, with the cooperation of those of us already born. A most serious social contract. Epic ramifications ahead. We know there is more to love than ritually giving birth. It matters what are the circumstances, what are the exigencies, what are the unglazed, unvarnished realities. Abortion means to redeem the time. We work to reduce unemployment to zero. Let us also conceive a stratagem that reduces the abortion rate to negligible. Life begins at contraception.

OUR BELIEFS, AND THE FACTS.

There is this singular, shocking, simple, seminal reality. Children need parents! We are no longer confused by the abortion debate. We are not debating our beliefs. We are debating children. We are not trying to belittle beliefs. We want to deal with the children. We believe adult women suffer immensely in abusive relationships. We also know this to be a fact. How much more would a baby suffer in an abusive relationship? Think of all the things we know for sure, and all the other things we believe. It seems clear. Many other people are wrong about what they believe. Some of us have to be talking rubbish, on purpose or in error. Many more of us are also wrong, about what we know for sure. How can these things logically be?

Both Sir Isaac Newton and Albert Einstein can't be right, in absolute terms, about the existence of relativity. Jesus Christ and Moses can't both be right, in absolute terms, about sin and law. Thankfully, we are not debating the speed of light, or salvation. In our debate, there are, however, the constants. Children need parents. Children are born into unknown events. Perhaps we need to stop saying, "I believe this, or I believe that". The list of beliefs seems gratuitously infinite. Maybe when in polite company, we need to say, "I can prove this, or I can prove that."

What an incredibly quiet world this would be.

Think gently about the bucket list of fondly held beliefs, now soundly debunked by nothing more invasive than empirical evidence. Let us start with the proverbial and oft-ridiculed flat earth belief. The "earth is the center of the universe." We know the stork brings mom her babies. We believe the hanged Saddam Hussein has his weapons of mass destruction hidden in Syria, not Iraq as we previously believed. In another billion years, we will find the missing link and prove evolution. President Kim Jong-un of North Korea is undoubtedly a powerful man. According to the Telegraph, 22nd May 2020. North Korea officially set the record straight. President Jong-un cannot bend space and time. Once upon a time, a British Prime Minister believed Adolf Hitler wanted peace in Europe. Dear Mr. Hitler even signed the historic Munich Agreement, to confirm the belief. In hindsight, all is clear and sublimely simple. A belief is not necessarily a fact.

Without reservation, however, beliefs are more fun. Beliefs are also much easier to believe than facts. The facts sometimes diverge with unapologetic abruptness, from our preferred reality. Using the same available information, we can still interpret and conclude differently. Many of us have looked at the same incident captured on tape, or read the same history, and arrived at quite different conclusions. We have our biases and our beliefs. Facts are a luxury when one tries to survive. It was safer not to believe in Jesus than not to believe in Comrade Stalin. Information easily gets distorted in its retelling. We should at least strive to have the facts, at the very least.

Take, for example, the varied interpretation of the well and universally known exploits of Christopher Columbus. Columbus came, he saw, and he kept a journal. Thank God. His narrative is consistent with our abortion discussion. Lots of lives, young and old, expired. The middle ages might still be aging without Columbus. He brought us to our bravest, newest incarnation of the Western world. Hard choices were an everyday reality for Admiral Christopher Columbus. Conditions were hostile and fluid, if not inherently toxic. Life and death. His or theirs. Columbus had to choose, and so do we. Christopher Columbus's effective suppression of the Amerindian Terrorist in 1492 could be a model for the present war on terror. Columbus organized a broad coalition of progressive nations against Arawak and Kalinago (Amerindian) insurgents and their black mercenary allies, the Moors. They had laid perennial siege to Portugal and Spain for most of the early fifteenth century.

It took the courageous rulers of Spain, Queen Isabella and King Ferdinand, to accept Columbus's relief proposal. Finally, Europe could take the fight to the Caribbean militants. Economically, Europe had been strangled, into dire economic and social straits, by the brutal and unrelenting incursion from overseas. Gold bullion disappeared as ransom, and as peace incentives, to Caribbean warlords. The Europeans paid reparation costs at a rate national treasuries could not hope to sustain. Aztec, Mayan, and Inca rulers hoarded most of that wealth in North and South America. Caribbean sponsored terror threatened to extinguish Europe, as a place viable for human habitation. There is no overstating, the immense political courage mobilized, to maintain the European response against the Caribbean threat. Captured Europeans, especially the Spanish soldiers, endured some of the most depraved conditions of imprisonment ever. Waterboarding involved being strapped unto a surfboard and dumped onto a coral reef. This was a siesta from the real mean, vile stuff.

To break the European resolve, the Caribbean terrorist set up special terror courts called Spanish Inquisitions. Especially notorious was the court at Guantanamo Bay, Cuba. Admiral Columbus, with the unwavering support of the huddled masses back home, sailed seas and slogged on the beaches. He sometimes retreated, but he never surrendered. Eventually, they won the fight, and a permanent peace installed. They left garrisons to serve and protect. The civilian population of the Caribbean he put back to work, expanding mining, tourism, and agriculture. The Caribbean economies soon flourished in legal trade.

Brave dedicated action, by Spanish marines, eventually resulted in the complete and permanent eradication of the terrorist threat from the Caribbean islands. Religious persecution of minorities, by human sacrifice obsessed Aztec priests, he abolished. Thank God for that. The victorious Spanish marines, for their dogged, determined defense of Europe, got christened Conquistadores. From Florida in the North to Peru in the South the Spanish shouldered, against all odds, the burden to save the civil way. Today, when we vacation in the Caribbean, we may wish to remember the sacrifice. The few who fought to secure the rights of the many. Visiting the Caribbean was not always a cruise or a holiday. Just ask the beleaguered heroes of 1492. Remember that Pina Colada we enjoy today started as a Bloody Mary. It may not be factual, but we can still believe in our story.

Part of the problem with the abortion discussion seems to be the narrow legal nature of the discussion. Yes, abortion is about killing life. This is definitive, and this is absolute. There is however a factual context to life, not just our beliefs. There is history. There is an imagined future. There is sociology. There is more to abortion than medical timelines & religious beliefs. We know children don't care for themselves. Children need parents. It appears there are more compartments to life than breathing.

The word torture is curious. When properly applied, no one should die. It is just wonderful to know. "No one died... they were just tortured." So we committed no murder that day? Jesus, it seems, surely was too broad with his definition of murder. Reality, for all known recorded history, has never had to ask for a second opinion. What was is. What happened, happened. What happens, happens. What is happening is happening. We know children not aborted are born. We know that aborted lives are dead and did not make it to childhood. We know abused children are here because someone insisted they be born. This is our reality. How we interpret these physical realities, creates our social realities of laws, taboos, and our belief systems.

Child protection services exist because we know unapologetic oppression afflicts the most vulnerable among us. In the world of facts, I beg to regard our beliefs as our personal and collective social recreation. When there is no abortion, a child is born. Then what? This seems to be a small, but a relevant question. A child is born. Then what? Our world view is most important to us. This does not change the facts. Reality is the self-existing, impartial narrative of what happens, even if we don't understand it. Reality is not what we prefer to believe happens. That we mislead ourselves is part of reality too. Imagine you offered an unconceived life, a childhood. Being a Christian, you would know this, "Through much trial and tribulation shall you inherit the kingdom of God." It would make sense to fast track the program. It is the will of God. We would try to get that child a black mom. One educated and not addicted to prescription or other drugs, and very beautiful with a cute pout. The father would be a handsome, hardworking, white gentleman raised to be the head of the home. What could go wrong?

The ages reveal a plurality of religious beliefs, a multiplicity of traditions, a wondrous variety in modes of governance, a riot in human imaginations. Of social inventions an infinity. Of cultures a veritable contradiction in grandeur. Of right and wrong, an endless diversity. We have long drawn our moral lines in the sand. As the flippancy of teenage angst would say, "Whatever!"

We should believe the truth. Then again, as we credit Pilate in asking Jesus Christ, "What is truth?" We have vested interests. As participants in our social experiments, we are self-calibrated to lie. This is where peer review can be helpful. Are we interested in children, or matters of sexual orthodoxy? We wish to regulate sexual behavior to the womb. Servitude is as natural as pregnancy. It is horrible to impose life on the unborn. Man is not born free. Man is born helpless. Humans like a good quarrel. One marinated, in every contentious irrelevance possible. Abortion supplies an inexhaustible supply for gossip and righteous indignation. When we discuss abortion, the basic issue is of life and death. This living and dying occurs in the environment we call our world. Who does not like a cute baby? No need to raise hands on this one. How do we create someone so they can be unwanted? Abortion is organically an honest issue. It lacks the manufactured complexion of the dress code debate. Should we wear miniskirts or burqas? Abortion is a legitimate issue of life, made infinitely more complex by social and religious dogma. We all know abortion is the earliest, but not the only way to kill, or torture a child.

A meaningful discussion of life yields to the context of life. As for death, the same applies. Context. Are you killing the guard at Auschwitz, or are you killing your server at the diner? Both provide poor service. As we know everybody has access to an opinion. Everybody does not have access, even to clean water, or a night's rest without medication. Everyone does not have access to their legs or brain. It is difficult to agree, to disagree. Riots break out over mere sports competitions. We ban, fine, and jail hooligans. Friendships succumb to devastating battles over baseball, basketball, hockey, football, cricket, and sex. It is not just a game after all. For abortion, there is no agreeing to disagree. It seems not good enough to say, "Okay, you go ahead have your baby, I'll kill mine". This leads to another war of words, "Is it yet really yet a baby, or a mass of actively dividing human cells?"

It sounds so inhumane. We wake in the morning, hopefully not in prison. We realize we have been in custody, since the days of our stunted youth. We are our cellmates, and our warden is the parliament. Society itself, of necessity, is a specie invasive to personal freedom. Power rules. Society can compel a woman to become a parent, just because it has the power too. Society can restrict a woman's childbearing to one child only, etc. etc. It has the power to. Society can decree that we conceive no new babies. Society can decree a minimum of five children per fertile female. It would all be legal. We are trying to figure out the reality of conception and childbirth. The law is secondary at this point. No matter what the laws say, children need parents. After birth, children will need caring for. These things we know.

For all our varied social mores and customs, mankind survives and sometimes thrives. There are regulations for everything. What to consume, where to consume it, with whom to consume it. Regulations govern every little ordinary, basic, simple, mundane matter like marriage, divorce, love, childbirth, and abortion. We know we are in prison because the granite legal walls surrounding us are so real. What of our vaunted personal freedoms? We possess only one. That is the will to choose. This is one tough and limited list of options.

For something as deadly as abortion, we would hope at the very least, the message we preach is true. Do we think we know the truth? How can we? What is the Rosetta stone of truth? What is the independent benchmark for truth? What is the scientific control for truth? Pilate may have said it best, "What in hell is truth?" True, he did not say hell according to the literature.

I love the Jewish God referred to in Isaiah 1:18. It reads, "Come now, let us reason together." Similarly, in Isaiah 41:2, "Produce your cause, says God; bring forward your strong case." As we can see a spirited debate is no new invention. The irony is. We have servants of the same God. They probably would never grant you an interview with their God, so you could debate your "heretical" views. Note to self. Always judge a God by his servants. I know we sometimes don't want to be reasonable. Reasonable takes us down a path we rightly fear treading. Where exactly will all this reasoning take us? Worst of all, where will it all end? Perfect love knows no fear. Love has no side deals to worry about.

The Founding Fathers (now the Founding Parents) of the United States found out the self-fulfilling nature of reason early on. "We hold these truths to be self-evident that all men are created equal that they are endowed by their Creator with certain unalienable Rights that among these are Life, Liberty, and the pursuit of Happiness." So they unanimously declared.

It was not long before the self-evident right to liberty ran into a dark little secret. The conflicts of logic are a very incon-

venient thing. The meeting to discuss liberty was pragmatic-
ally and duly adjourned, to a time more commodious, for the
pursuit of universal happiness. A civil war, two world wars,
and many misadventures later, we are still reading the minute
papers on race relations. George Orwell in his novella 'Animal
Farm' solved the conundrum. He declared all equal, but some
to be more equal than others. This makes perfect present sense.
Our vested interests make honest debate an oxymoron.

For eons, humans have worshiped at nature's altar. The god
of the sun, the moon, the stars, the ox, the serpent, the sea,
the river, the blue pebble, and the flawless diamond. The mum-
mified Pharaoh is Ra, the dagger pierced Julius Caesar joins the
pantheon of Roman gods. I dare one of us to tell the Pharaoh
he is not Ra incarnate. Go ahead. Make Pharaoh's intolerant day.
Weighing in from the Far East, The Buddha finds, in all the confusion of life, a venerable middle way. Before his time, the potent
Vedas of the Hindu would have transported the patient peni-
tent to (Moksha) Nirvana. From the disputed Judean capital,
Jerusalem, a crucified Jesus Christ conquers the reality of death,
with the reality of the resurrection. A one true God, and final
Prophet sprouts and blossoms into Islam in the barren Arabian
Desert. In the Celestial land, the descendants of Confucian vir-
tue switch allegiance to a new Communist gold standard. The
United States of American begins the worship of Prohibition.
While the sage minds of Socrates' Greece sacrificed to Zeus and
Hera, the modern intellectual elite finds comfort in the pleas-
ures of atheism.

There are so many beliefs, so many persuasions, so many
personal realities, so many people to please. It would exhaust
a human lifetime to study, or cater to them all. There are
multiple billion brains, all washed in the purity of their social banners. The banners of Islam, of Hinduism, of Agnosticism, of Paganism, of Socialism, of Communism, of Capitalism,
of Apathy, of Agnosticism, of Ancestor worship, of Hedonism,
of Protestant Christianity, of Catholicism, of faithlessness, of
ignorance and democracy. Surely these divergent seas of be-

lievers, and non-believers, can't be all right. There is only one earth we occupy. Different time zones, and Divine legislation, but still one globe. Maybe we are all wrong.

The sun still shines, regardless of our beliefs, and heedless of how much we love darkness. It seems hopeless to expect a reasoned discourse, when dogma is the first offense, and sometimes the only line of defense. Of what sincere use is a belief forcibly inserted into our brain? We may as well insert beliefs via Meth or Crack pipe. It is simple. If we make a public declaration, we should want them dissected and examined. Unless our aim is basically to deceive and conquer. Religious folks especially, should stop with the blasphemy defense. Accept that if you preach, you are ready to debate. If the books of Moses command the death of all Canaanites nearby, then it does. All means male and female, babe and suckling, and the unborn too. These bylaws for holocaust came after the Israelites received their Constitution, the Ten Commandments.

One commandment according to our modern Bible commanded, "Thou shalt not kill." The same inspired word commanded thus about murder. Numbers 36.3, "So you shall not pollute the land you dwell in. For blood it defiles the land and the land cannot be cleansed of the blood shed in it, but by the blood of him that shed it. We now see killing made a moral and civic duty by the very same God.

Inquiry is contrary to sound business, as we want paying subscribers, not honest investigators. Believe this, accept that, No examination necessary. New, improved revelation, made for immediate consumption. Don't add your brain. For all the vast stocks of varied beliefs, sincere and otherwise. For all our myriad social interpretations, humankind has lived and died with routine predictability. Regardless of our beliefs, the human corpses keep piling up, generations without end. Heedless of our wishes and our desires, the day comes and reduces all to a state of death. So far this has been the unedited, predictable human experience.

Death: no killing required. Life: love and care required. In the spirit of peace, let us invite ourselves to a reasoned debate. While we still live, while concepts and notions persist, while social constructs still are of relevance. While our society still permits free speech, let us debate. Inordinate repetition proves we can die and we die. That small window of life continues to make for scintillating historical drama. Eternal consequences await some affirm. Jesus claims to have gone there and come back. All in three days.

Where two or three gather, human society comes to birth. Our personal decisions now become tools of collateral damage or collateral benefit. Tools of progress, or weapons of mass destruction. Before the great religions of our time came into being, human beings still had to synthesize modes of communal conduct and social behavior. The protestant churches we attend are tenderloins, in the religious scheme of things. We all know of Mr. John Calvin, and Martin Luther, not King this time. We know of Anglican King Henry the 8th. Henry the Eighth is notable. King Henry created his Church of England because he needed to abort a marriage, and the Catholic Pope would not allow him. Practical fellow, this King Henry.

The Protestants, thankfully, came to sanction contraception as morally acceptable at the 1930 Seventh Lambeth Conference. Freedom of conscience helps us to live our lives as we think best. The law may not always approve. God could have forced us to love one another. God could have made us his obedient pets, dutifully doing as we were told. God could have forced us to have children too. God wants to feel special, like we gratefully enjoy his company. He wants us to choose him.

I think we have misunderstood a little bit how blessings work. The blessing does not do the chore or activity. The blessing promises success in the endeavor. Our agricultural enterprise can be blessed or cursed. Our childbearing can be blessed or cursed. This was clearly explained to the Israelites ready to enter the promised land. The deed belongs to the doer. The blessing prospers the doer and the deed. The doing activates the blessing if God agrees. As per the Genesis record. The blessing of the Tree of Life existed simultaneously with the curse of the Tree of the Knowledge of Good and Evil. Eve's choice, shared by Adam activated the curse. Having a child is not a blessing or a curse. It is a choice we better wish is blessed. Have mercy and careful thought with the reproductive privilege. Life begins at contraception. Even when your employer won't include it in the health insurance package.

Life existed before human religion. If life came before religion, the ills of mankind are essentially the ills of human nature, and not of a specific religious orthodoxy. Examine any of the purges finessed by the Communist Soviet Union and then tell us which church the Politburo attended? We will not discuss the People's Republic of China, because that would constitute interference in their internal affairs. As the ancient Uighur and Tibetan proverbs say, "A bad idea to say the least."Religion does not need an Eternal God, just a supreme leader is enough. The important denominator is the power to enforce conformity. Philosophy as a means of social control is clear in religious worship. We should remember though that before the religion was the man. Our beliefs conveniently, or otherwise, bow to the mind of the superior deity or deities. Life itself obliges us to decide and to choose. Yes, we should choose what is good.

Is it good to create persons to hurt them? Is it good to create persons, to have them abandoned and neglected? Is it good to make small mistakes, bigger mistakes? Is it good to make mistakes at all? Is it good to compel others to inherit our mistakes? Look at all the curiosities man has fashioned for our service. We use cutting instruments for agriculture or a sneak assault on our neighbor. A Viking ax could fell timber for a home. The ax could also, unceremoniously, usher an English monk to St Peter's pearly gates. We don't need the National Rifle Association to convince us our guns don't kill, we can worship our pistols if we please. The fact remains, we first produced the rifle. The rifle did not produce us. We consume ourselves with our very inventions, both social & material.

We should wonder aloud. It's always a valid question. To

what good will we put that ax, or gun, money, cellphone, or our burgeoning pregnancy? The philosophies of our religions, secular or otherwise, once offered for public consumption, should be open to rigorous social exam. If we preach, it seems unfair to silence the critics by yelling, " Unpatriotic, treason, blasphemy."

Judaism, Christianity, and Islam, in that pecking order, are relatively youthful social indoctrination programs. I think this is a good observation for the abortion question. The world existed and functioned, or was dysfunctional for generations, without the present codified enlightened revelations. The Bible, of the Jews and Christians, shows the concept of morality existed before God etched the Ten Commandments in stone on Mount Sinai. Jesus distilled morality to an insipid, "Do unto others as you would want for yourself." Brilliant stuff. As for me. I am just dying to be born to parents who don't feel ready for my birth.

Why are we fighting? We are at war for the Motherland, for the Fatherland, for Democracy, for freedom, for our country, for our families, for religions, for our Gods. Never are we in a fight, because of our wounded pride, or we envy our neighbor, or we covet their goods. It has always been convenient to influence one another by stamping our cause, "Made in Heaven." The morality which condemns abortion is duty-bound to flourish, not expire, after childbirth. The children are forlornly awaiting the proof of the love pudding. Consider the vaunted sanctity of life. Life is sacred, as long as it remains housed in the womb. Oh, the palpable, if not the audible disappointment. That sacred pregnancy produced a mere girl. Nine whole months wasted. Idea! We can sell her. People always are looking for pretty virgins to buy.

The secular religions of greed and ambition have for eons governed us. Our religions have spawned social upheaval and cataclysm with generational punctuality. The two most recent world wars in our history had little to do with making the world safe for babies and pregnant women. Julius Caesar's bloody subjugation of Gaul, as boasted by the god himself, had little to do with any perceived slights or blasphemies against Jupiter or Janus. It was a simple case of a man doing what a man thought he wanted to do. Our lives will not be any more secure without religion. Man is religion. Man is the custodian of his religion and his reasoning. Illogic, by whatever name, is still illogical. Greed, whatever its banner is still greed.

We have all our vested interests in the dividends of error. The question is, "Do we want to be reasonable today?" In the beginning, there was no abortion. Soon after the beginning, there was procreation. It is easy to see, without the business of procreation, there is no matter of abortion. Abortion is avoidable, rather easily. No fertilization. No abortion. No insemination, no conception, no pregnancy. Rudimentary stuff.

Finally, at least once in the history of humankind, here is one thing we can all agree on. No fertilization equals no abortion. There is no proverbial chicken and egg dilemma. We can't abort what we don't have. The pro-choice lobby might want to appreciate this simple fact. Yes, we should be relentlessly active, concerning the secondary status of women. This power imbalance can greatly affect their authority to regulate their fertilities. I know enough women who had tubal ligations only because the doctor's authority overawed that of the husband. Life begins at contraception.

So where do babies come from? We assume babies come because parents want to become parents. Women don't become pregnant, because it's an inevitable part of the menstrual cycle. Procreation is forced, or it is the voluntary indulgence in the naughty act. Our views on sexual activity, as an approved recreation, may be the real cornerstone in this abortion business. We know there is a global obsession with sex. There is even a prehistorically coined term, "sexual immorality," still in active circulation. It has proven very difficult to deal with the realities of abortion, because of our complicated views on sex. Alas, human living is mainly about dealing with things avoidable... and with things unavoidable. Today, there are births many, miscarriages likely, and abortions surely. As long as there is no intercourse of things male and female there is no material basis for abortion. Abortion is a social construct, not a naturally occurring biological inevitability.

In this our twenty-first century, the word abortion connotes premeditated, not accidental death. We will die because we exist. Just that minor defect of an existence condemns us all to death. An inevitable death has been the most strident and punctual testimonial in human history. Birth. As long as children have unwilling parents, there exists a prima facie, socially inherent, humanely urgent need for abortion. It is a very simple moral matter. Abortion is a reasonable civic duty, which unfortunately involves death. We are taking you off life support before you are born. So no, abortion is not murder, and no abortion is not a woman's inalienable natural right. Abortion is not a fun moment. As Jesus astutely observes, neither is life "It had been better for that man if he had never been born."

From a purely biological standpoint, abortion is no big deal. The unborn contributed zero resources in its conception. This sperm and egg remain separate, as we know, unless people fool around. Fool around is quite literal in this context. The fertilized egg, now the single-celled zygote, divides and forms into more cells called a blastocyst. This person travels from the fallopian tubes and attaches to the woman's uterus to establish a blood supply. Pregnancy has now occurred. This is from conception to pregnancy. I am saying all of this to point out we are not immediately pregnant upon conception. Neither, the woman nor the person attached to the uterus, knows this magnificent scientific breakthrough has occurred. This is the person the morning-after pill would have killed, as pregnancy would not occur. If this were a bank heist, we would have robbed the armored trucks carrying the cash en route, before it made it to the bank.

So several days after we had unprotected sex we are pregnant. The placenta and umbilical cord will form and we will not get our period. The cash is safely inside the bank vault. Now mifepristone also known as RU-486 or the abortion pill is used to kill this newly attached human being from the womb. Pregnancies go from ground zero to nine months.

To understand what happened to the person just born, all we have to do is ask. After the baby is born we debrief them about the details of their miraculous and sacred journey. That baby, not wanting to disappoint, cries, and does not stop for a few months following. They are telling us we just don't understand. Two years later, still no details of the incredible journey. Five years later that baby can speak and scream curses. Still no details. Twenty- five years later that baby is writing, with authority in medical journals, about the thoughts and aspirations of other fetuses. The fact is. Babies can't be more complex, more aware, or more mature in the womb than when we receive them outside. We have an unbroken chain of custody. Having performed so many abortions, we know a bit about the physical stages of human pregnancy. We know this without a doubt.

Abortion denies no unborn child any material property, or intellectual ambition. They are born lacking both. You have aborted no dream, or scheme the baby was feverishly trying to finish before delivery. Remember we have many newborn babies in our possession. They come out hungry and cold. We usually provide help. This is exactly what we have been waiting for nine months to do. Fetuses need parents not only birth. The newborn human person testifies to the mental condition of the fetus. At its most developed, a baby is blissfully alive but ignorant. No one is denying the unborn stimuli. They are unaware of the intricacies of their birth. We impose our humanity on our pregnancies. We buy what we think they would like for the nursery. We name them what we think would be interesting. We baptize and circumcise them because we think they will appreciate it. The life we claim to deny the unborn has not yet started, except in our minds, and our desires. This is the indisputable evidence validated by childbirth itself.

A woman spends nine months nurturing a pregnancy. Naturally, and strategically, she wants no harm to come to her unborn darling. It is very frightening to hear about abortion then. When we crush the skull of a fetus, we are imposing our appreciation for cruelty and brutality. If we did this to a rat just to see it writhe in pain, our friends would start thinking of Ted Bundy and other psychopaths. It is our common human destiny, not our common human maturity, which binds us to the unborn. We know they are only a few cells large, and unaware of their existence. We love them. They are our family, our very genetic material. They are our protected specie.

For many Christians, God gave humans not a mission to procreate family, but a direct command. Be fruitful and multiply. It is very convenient to deal with Gods who publish. See Genesis 1:28. In the Genesis narrative, it is clear. God issued his famous blessing on multiplication before the well-known fall of mankind. Focus on the word blessed. It would be reasonably irresponsible of God to ask an evil Adam and Eve to produce babies for him. God did not even think them nice enough to remain in the suburban paradise he called Eden. He expelled mankind to the ghetto, to rough it out. We know you don't ask your drunk friend to pick up your wife from the airport. Poor example. We know you don't ask your drunk friend to pick up your kids from school. We do these things responsibly.

I cannot see the blessing of being born already high. The prophet Jeremiah had a few thoughts on birth himself, "Why did I leave the womb to see labor and sorrow, that my days should be consumed with shame?" Our authorization is to reproduce nothing but joy and blessings.

We see God adapting his policies to suit the current situation. New circumstances, new decisions. In the beginning, both man and beast ate vegetable matter, for example. I think we can also agree the earth was very empty then. The first census came up with only two people. In another event, God aborted his entire human creation, including the unborn babies and toddlers in a great flood. Afterward, God blessed Noah and children, telling them to repopulate the empty earth. With God, reproduction is a family blessing. A gift, not a command of coercion. How does reproduction itself become a moral duty? Where is the blessing? The devil himself is busy in the business of reproduction. There are children of God and children of the Devil. For God's sake, Satan has more children than God. Does this make him obedient? John 8:44, Jesus says to the unbelieving Jews, "You are of your father the devil." Talk about anti-Semitism. Be fruitful and multiply," who says Satan does not obey God?

There are instructions to tend the garden and to have dominion over the beast of the earth. This means, if we don't have a few animals personally in subjection, we have failed to obey a very clear and ancient directive. That God permits miscarriages makes you wonder. Has God forgotten his previous reproductive prescription? Be fruitful and multiply.

Let us head to more reasonable questions, like why don't we marry our brothers and sisters like Cain and his siblings? Or even like Abraham and his half-sister Sarah? It is written so it shall be done. "By the sweat of your brow, you shall eat bread." Please stop cheating by using air-conditioning. No room for slaves in that command. The holy observers must appreciate the language of Genesis, where the story all begins. God said to the woman, "I will greatly multiply thy sorrow and your conception; in sorrow, you shalt give birth to children." "In sorrow." I know no other definition of sorrow than sorrow. Interestingly, he does not say the children would be born into sorrow. God does not stop there. He tells the fruit-loving Eve "your desire shall be to your husband." This not so awful if you are the husband, but God continues, "and he shall rule over you."

What we see here is a drastic change in a woman's lot in life. A female now becomes vulnerable because of her reproductive talents. She is also liable to be subject to her male friend. That's what the Genesis narrative says. Reproduction makes a woman at least as vulnerable as a snake that just swallowed a big meal. She had better have a real loving, all righteous, all-knowing husband. She would be fine with one like Jesus, the second Adam, to rule her over and impregnate her. As we know from Revelation, a woman in great sorrow gave birth to a ruler prince. This is entirely another story, so for another time maybe.

We can safely deduce that before the fruit-eating incident, Adam did not rule over Eve, nor was she supposed to have a near-death encounter during pregnancy and delivery. Neither was she supposed to expect pregnancy on a monthly cycle. It appears very safe to conclude that God never intended Eve to single-handedly populate the earth, hence her new potential, to have greatly increased reproductive capacities. Every pregnancy made Eve vulnerable. Ladies and gentlemen, our job as believers, would be to ask God for a better deal, because as Jesus said, "In the beginning, it was not so." Life begins at contraception. At least, for women and children, it does.

It is not insignificant that Jesus failed to leave a few holy children behind. We know Mary, her sister Martha, and Mary Magdalene loved him to death and beyond. Jesus skipped the marriage and procreation and moved straight into creating spiritual babies. Then he says, "Many are called, few are chosen." It sounds so much like abortion. Let the record show: Jesus, the perfect man, bailed on marriage and kids.

It is natural to procreate, we may say. Death holds itself as a paramount testimony in all things natural. Nature teaches many lessons. It is up to us to learn the lessons we think relevant. Surely there are natural lessons of females consuming or "abandoning" their young. Turtles have no moms waiting to cuddle them. No one to teach them the mysteries of the seas. You are born, you are on your own. These are natural lessons. The current libel is of praying mantis females consuming their mates after copulation. Recycling at its best. There is overwhelming evidence of rampant sexual promiscuity in nature. Where there are two or more male dogs, it's possible some natural display of homosexual behavior. Dogs certainly like cunnilingus. How natural.

The dear Penguins of the South Pole naturally teach how parents can share the joys of raising the young, and of putting food on the table. The ostrich shows you can hatch your brood in the wide, uncaring open. They also show how both parents cooperate with the baby work, as the males also help incubate the eggs. Sea turtles naturally teach moms to travel overseas to have anchor babies. Nature teaches survival of the fittest. Contrary to PETA doctrine, nature teaches meat is fine if you like it. No social campaign will put the lioness off her meat. Nature teaches communal living and group security. Nature teaches drought, nature teaches flood, nature also teaches rain in moderation. Nature teaches violence, nature teaches cooperation. Nature teaches survival of the fittest. Nature teaches many lessons, mankind learns what we wish. Nature teaches times and seasons. Children need parents before birth. Life begins at contraception.

SERIAL KILLERS.

Let's continue, before the civil bickering starts. What is right and what is wrong? I hope we agree on one other petty thing. Abortion is about the death of a growing human life. If it is not alive, why kill? Abortion is not the evaluation of the dogmas of particular religions, or tray groups. Children need parents. This is the question on everyone's lips. "What about the dear babies?" This is what every legislator wants to know about, even before asking, "Where are the taxes coming from?"

Some of us cannot imagine life without abortion. We call ourselves Pro-choice. Almost as a reflex action, the sight of coat hangers, Pro-lifers, back alleyways, or convicted abortionist, Kermit Gosnell's clinics, cause us an acute anguish. Abortion we extol, as a basic and fundamental human-female right. We promote the virtues of a well-lit, competently staffed, sterile clinic. An abortion clinic is, to us, what the Statue of Liberty once symbolized to immigrants and refugees. This, in brief, is Pro-choice. Others passionately oppose abortion. We call ourselves Pro-life. For Pro-lifers, abortion is murder. For some, abortion because of incest, and an endangered mother's life is pardonable, but it is most regrettable. Abortion remains for us, the domain of licensed and unlicensed serial killers. Even more briefly, this is Pro-life.

Debate rages. Misery and pain grow obese. Female bellies continue to blossom with the promise of fetal fruit. Debate consumes the land and mind. Legislatures balance what is so-cial, against what is scientific and what is moral, against what is politically expedient. Can the courts provide the unborn the ruling which is both morally and legally tenable? Religion preaches and prays in near-global solidarity against the bane of child destruction. Women cry about the baby they would love to deliver, but can't keep. Abortion remains.

Contraception is promoted. Contraception is condemned. Adoption is recommended. Child abuse continues to shrug off and muscle away the molestations of love and restraint. The statistics are appalling. Rescues are staged. Courts are picketed. Lobbyist lobby. Fees are paid and pocketed, large and small. Abortion remains. For now, abortion remains. The pro-choice are deadly eager to save their beloved procedure. The pro-life breathe to secure abortion's death. Abortion is not a twentieth-century creation. For eons, the enterprising and the desperate have purged the unborn from the body, though not necessarily from the conscience. The Roman poet Juvenal, of ancient fame, leaves us a metered testimony to this effect, "How powerful the drugs, how subtle the skill of the abortionist, paid to murder mankind within the womb" Today, we can add, "How modern the clinic." Juvenal was not exactly pleased. Some Roman ma-trons just wanted to have fun, commit adultery, all without maternal consequence. Juvenal seemed to have little problem with the unbridled blood orgies of the gladiatorial games, just with women gladiators. The ancients also used contraception. Rome, it is reported, used the plant Silphium to extinction. It prevented pregnancy and also induced medical abortions. It is amazing how every generation believes it invented the earth, society, and notions of freedom, and moral debates.

Pro-choice visionaries expect universal abortion suffrage. From pole to pole, the elevation of the abortion practice is craved. An elevation from covert to overt. An elevation from government-harassed, to government-sanctioned and subsid-ized even. Economies contract, inflation is on the rise, salaries are seemingly eternally on the freeze. At a time such as this, the female midsection expands. Some are happy about it. Some fly into a suicidal panic. Some visit the local abortion clinic. Some take a trip. Some do discreet structural adjustments, thanks to their sympathetic gynecologist. Some die. Some grin and bear it.

Abortion remains an issue of death. When there is a sperm spill in the vaginal ocean, Parenthood looms into significance. Life or death? That is the question. Abortion is one of the great wonders of the modern world. Politicians wonder, "Why the hell did this have to come up during my term?" The pro-life wonder, "Why don't they bring the baby to term. Do they want to go the hell?" The pro-choice wonder, "Why don't these pro-lifers all go to hell?" The greatest wonder about abortion. Can the embryo or fetus wonder at all?

In a good year, according to the World Health Organization, about 40-50 million abortions are performed. This logs in at 125,000 abortions per day. In that same good year, we expect about 130 million births according to the United Nations. This is approximately 360,000 babies per day. Allow for gross statistical error, but still, it is obvious large numbers of persons give birth and more than a statistically insignificant few abort. Depending on who you are, either or both figures can be positively, nay negatively horrible.

The birth figures translate into 360,000 well prepared and equipped parents. They smile in joy as they welcome the long-awaited birth of their children. We won't mention the thousands of siblings just hungry to see that cute new, baby mouth at the breakfast table. Contraception for me is not mainly about regulating the number of children. The critical value of contraception is regulating when you wish to become a parent. It will take eighteen years to raise that one child you don't want, anyway.

The question remains, and at that, unanswered. The abortion question is no rhetorical one. Is it fair to a fertilized egg, an embryo, or a fetus, to condone or practice abortion? The next question is this. Is it fair to make the unborn born? Lovemaking is natural, we should do it any time, and anywhere. It's good, let's do it. I don't see us thinking of the unborn as a person. I don't see us considering the unborn as an individual. I don't see us understanding that children inherit themselves, eventually. I get the impression children are things to be born because they are here. It seems like a not intelligent plan. I see us obsessed with the control of the adult person and their sexuality.

Remember, when Satan encouraged Jesus if he was the Son of God to jump from a pinnacle of the Temple. Jesus had a written guarantee from Psalm 91:12 that the angels of God would keep him safe and not even allow him to stub his toe. If any person had too much health insurance coverage, it would be Jesus Christ. Jesus told the tempting devil, "It is also written, you shalt not tempt the Lord your God."

There is a time for everything and every purpose. Forget for a moment fetal viability. We remember always parental viability. The pro-life. Are we sexist, sentimental sillies, determined to deny a woman control over her womb? Those who vacillate with the winds of circumstance is our case-by-case approach the way to go? Pro-choice. Are we rabid hell-bent fiends? Our mouths foaming pain and hurtful death? Is our one purpose, to destroy and devour unborn life so we can indulge our sexual debauchery?

In 1973, the Supreme Court of the United States legalized abortion. The decision to abort in the approximately first three months of pregnancy (first trimester) became the de facto, exclusive preserve of the pregnant female and her doctor. For the second and third trimesters, with increased fetal viability, the states ostensibly, for a love for life, could regulate abortion, providing the life or health of the mother was not at stake. Largely, the decision received a cordial welcome. Since Roe v. Wade, however, we have been wading in an abortion quagmire. Abortion is legal Vietnam.

Today, an acid pro-life environment is ceaselessly lashing the landmark decision. The aim is to prove Roe v. Wade is founded not upon the unshakeable, solid rock of constitutional jurisprudence. But it was conceived upon a porous and readily eroded limestone of social accommodation. There is fear playing the Supreme Court trump card could make abortion a severely compromised legal right. These days, psychologically at least, this erosion has nearly reduced legal abortion to a censored activity. The right to an abortion in the USA seems to be more of a grudging compromise, in a pluralistic society, than a true constitutional right.

In the Planned Parenthood v. Casey, (1999 remix of the U.S Supreme Court's, 1973 hit single Roe v. Wade), the court asserted the rights of the State to regulate with reason abortion, in the previously sacrosanct first trimester. The face of abortion on demand, at that moment, lost its self-assured smirk of being above state law. Under the 1973 ruling, by the time the State had jurisdiction to express its interest in the fate of the unborn, we would have performed many an abortion in that first-trimester window.

Some, impatient with the continued upholding of Roe v. Wade by the courts, wish to reformat abortion rights. Popular politics, instead of robed judges, would decide it. All this takes is an overturning of Roe v. Wade. Perhaps abortion needs its specific constitutional amendment. "And the right of women not to bear shall not be infringed."

Abortion is a legal issue larger than life. Abortion either is or is not murder, or abortion sometimes is murder or abortion may not be about murder. Abortion may be about the childhood prospects for the unborn. Abortion may be about persons becoming reluctant parents. A court can only interpret the laws provided. Children need willing parental care. No law or the lack of law can change this. Perhaps life starts at contraception.

One American export staunchly resisted in the Caribbean is abortion. English Caribbean law usually assures that all attempts to procure or facilitate an abortion be held in legal and social contempt. Caribbean women are not formally interfered with for going overseas to perform the taboo deed. Access to abortion is much less available than access to marijuana. If no one dies, little legal reaction so far follows, but some social recrimination may be inevitable. Very few people don't mind being called, "A walking cemetery."

The legal justification for the 1973 abortion charter espouses the trimester framework and personal rights to privacy. The court has since replaced the trimester concept with the viability framework. For some, the reasoning remains, if the fetus cannot survive outside the mother, then abortion is permissible. We concede knowledge, interpretations, and technology are perpetually in flux. We are not aborting trimesters. We are interrupting human growth to viability and beyond. An abortion aims to stop the baby from being viable at the earliest.

Abortion season is mainly during the first trimester. The risks are low... for the woman. The unborn is much easier to kill, as we would expect. Medical abortions, with pills, but not the morning-after pill, take place within the first ten weeks. This makes the procedure easier and cheaper, and very safe for the woman. We can't say, mother. The more we delay an abortion, the more we put a child in danger of being born. Our delays conspire to force a child to be born unwanted. Viability is nature's uncompromised testimony that Parents must prepare for birth.

The pro-life are adamant that more than a few take abortion to pregnancy's very edge, and beyond the edge even. Whether it is by abortion, or by giving birth, we would not want a culture of child abuse. We all have a human right to show love for one another. It is our choice.

One of the new additions to the abortion debate is the old concept of life beginning at conception. This view became official Catholic doctrine in 1869 when infallible Pope Pius IX decreed the human soul is born at conception. It is not only maintained that the life of a human being begins at conception. We are besides assured we have a human being at conception. Just a very microscopic one. We intend this arrangement to deny abortionists any grace period in which to ply the trade. We fixate on law and murder. We forget the unborn inherit what we sow.

The uninitiated often think of abortion as an ongoing debate. It is not. The noise we hear is from two opponents more ideologically divorced than Capitalism and Communism ever were. There is no debate, just the loud presentation of opposing views. As far as the pro-life and pro-choice camps agree, there is little left to talk about. The battles rage in teenage minds and the main casualty is unborn life. We must occasionally call a truce. It is civilized. We should abandon our fixed Western Front positions, and in good faith reassess our lines of reasoning.

We know from scientific experience the microscopic beginnings of human beings. We know sperm and eggs develop into human beings. Assured are we of the human life locked within the chromosomes. So, it is obvious to us all. A human being exists at conception. It should be no great feat to locate that very obvious human being. We all know this without question. A parent must exist after conception. We demand the parent be a willing one.

The solution to the abortion question cannot die waiting. When will new scientific knowledge show us, at precisely what point we have a human being? We know religion already, knows when we have a human being. A cave person should be able to deal with abortion with as much competence as a modern doctor of science. Those with no access to, or interest in, the great discoveries of modern science, must still make moral decisions. We should take pains to rely on rational thought and common observation. Cave people figured out the breast milk was for the baby and the breast for fondling. The basis of the Golden rule is this. Keep it simple. This is so, as all can't fact check the statistical or research data.

A human being can be a live human being or a dead human being. A human being can be a developed human being, or a developing human being, or a future human being. The fact birth is a process, does not deny a life his or her humanity. It confirms it. Human life is a unique, patented process. Human life is a process, not a onetime endgame. We know this. It has to start sometime, somewhere. Therefore, we abort the process. We are certain of the outcome. Human experience taught us that. Life itself commands the process of development. Life is not a mechanical process of manufacture. Life is genetically pre-determined. The ingredients used to make a human being are specifically and automatically coded to create a human being. Fertilize and voila. Abortion is a race against the inevitability of giving birth to a human being. Abortion is war against human maturity. Maybe we are confusing human self-awareness with human status itself. Even a corpse is a dead human being.

We are sure of the results. We know when the results are strange. Remember the black couple with the white baby. From the vantage of mature adulthood, we can make an honest con-clusion. The end product was the product, although not always fully manifested. A human being can be a zygote, an embryo, a fetus, or any other classification we may wish. It had to start human to finish human. A woman expects a baby, not a pet cat, at the end of her pregnancy.

That the Virgin Mary asked, "How can these things be, as I have not had intercourse," tells. Most people used to know that keeping men and women apart would cause zero new births. The developing life is unique to human life. There can be no contention about that. The reality remains. Even if all are equally human, all humans are not equally mature, equally de-veloped, equally aware, or equally conscious. I don't think we should force an artificial debate about fetal humanity. There is human life, and there is the process of human maturity. Just like building Notre Dame Cathedral was not in one day, although Rome was.

We evolve from just this to all that. One day we are young and foolish. A few years later we are older and more foolish. It pays to regard human life does not equal conscious human life. Additionally, a "human being" is not always conscious of its humanity. Those of us who are conscious think for those in a coma, or who are just sound asleep. When a human being dies the consciousness exits the scene, yet human life still inhabits the corpse for a time. The heart, and the liver, kidneys, are kept alive, in the hope of an organ transplant. Even with cardiac deaths, living human tissue is harvested. The tissue is alive, and it has all the human DNA. A freshly severed human head can have tissue harvested from it. Is that chromosome laden head a human being? This human being has lost its being. It is unaware of its status. It has no appreciation for its present tense. It is amazing to see what tricks beheaded poultry are capable of.

A fertilized egg has come into being. It is patently unaware of its "being" status. It relies on us to expect it. Before we got so smart, we knew the quickening was not at conception. Long ago, God destroyed Sodom and Gomorrah, and a few other wicked cities. We know the story of self-indulgence, unbridled pride, self-service, and sodomy. I note, God did not arrange adoptive parents for the unborn children. Could it be the unborn were entertaining deviant sexual thoughts while in utero? Saint Paul, in Romans 9:10, has this to say about unborn morality, "But when Rebecca also had conceived by one, even our father Isaac. For the children being not yet born, neither having done any good or evil." Humanity is a process, and our humanity has consequences. Eternally. Jesus chose his words carefully. "Unless you be born again, you cannot see the Kingdom of God." When we are born there are parents awaiting our deliverance. It is important to see, in the Jesus Christ scenario of birth, you get to choose if you wish to be born again. We accept and choose to be imprisoned, and tortured, and killed for the name of our Savior. Critically, our new father never leaves us nor forsakes us.

The abortion battle remains serious and fetus wrenching. I find it expedient to accept a freshly fertilized egg as a human being. I find it convenient to concede an implanted egg, one week old, to be a human being. It remains that our human being must still develop in stages and phases, just as we all do. Can you imagine appreciating, from conception, you are very much unwanted? Worst of all, imagine you are Rebecca's son Esau. From conception, you know Jacob I have loved Esau I have hated. I'm sure the unborn know, but being pro-life they don't care. They just want to be born. Dad is in jail for raping mom, but that's just because mom did not marry dad. Anyway, who needs parents? Who even needs a normal brain? Deformity? What deformity? It's just the inside that matters. Get out of here.

Fetal viability is only a small bit of the abortion equation. There is the after birth to deal with. Pregnancy shows how unborn life manually ties itself to the female. From the very womb, children do not grow and fed themselves. Reality never evades. Children continue to need willing parents. Our word games are of no help to the world's grieving young. The pain of giving birth has long ceased for the mother. Birth pangs beckon the child's new dawn.

Our awareness of self confirms a process of growth and death. Perhaps the more we appreciate the humanity of the unborn, the more compliant our minds will be to their unborn situation. It is a certain truth all alive today, and all dead yesterday, at one time wore the designation unborn. It does not matter how we label the unborn. Any human being is free to define another human being at his or her leisure. Children need willing parents. We start their lives at contraception.

The unborn are very ineffective at lobbying for their very survival. They kick at us, and all we do is giggle. They give us morning sickness and we grimace and take it in stride. We impose our life decisions on the unborn. We must depart from pretending that a first-trimester pregnancy favors an abortion, and a near viability pregnancy grudgingly succumbs to abortion. A first-trimester abortion is evidently more convenient. We abort the unborn because we want to. It is not the trimesters, which make us do it. It is not viability or non-viability who has abortions. We make the choices we prefer. We explain these choices with the aid of word labels, like human and viable. Time has connotations, and time has consequences. Abortion battles urgently against time. This time abortion law must unambiguously safeguard. Abortion is a sexually transmitted disease. Contraception will cure abortion.

Life does not automatically create decisions for us. For example, when we hear of a flood. We know warning lades the word flood. Flood means, "Destruction flows, get the sandbags ready and run." The flood will always be a flood and behave like a flood. What decisions we make about the flood, or how we interpret flooding, is entirely up to us. The phrase "human being at conception" means here is a human being. We must now decide about our relationship with him or her. Heedless of whether we are pro-life or pro-choice, babies need care. Regardless of words like viable or non-viable. Fertilized eggs, not aborted, grow to be born into mature adults. We have billions of case studies to validate this position. Conception does not produce love, or family, or care, or holiness. We also have billions of case studies to validate this position.

It is illogical to use our very definition of what is a human being, to justify our treatment of unborn life. Children need parents, end of the story. Children don't just need to be born. Miscarriages of logic can be devastating for some. Definition yields social response. Words evoke deeds. We know you don't yell fire in a crowded place as an April fool's joke.

The blacks, enslaved by divine right, were color branded to sub-humanity among other little indiscretions. Would a slave woman, be immoral, if she chose not to bear her child, into the privileged society of plantation slavery? Black slaves, in the American South, were a quarter of a full human being. A black fetus would be practically non-human. Perfect abortion bait. He or she still would become a fine slave though. Oh, how our religious and social views have evolved. Name-calling is not idle. Is abortion murder? The murder name-calling distracts us from actual family responsibilities. One thing remains the same, children still need parents. Whether it is the she-wolf of Romulus and Remus or Kipling's Mowgli, children need parents. Banning abortion does not manufacture parents.

What needs accurate classification in this deadly business of abortion, are our motives, intentions, and purposes. What demands accurate labeling are our attitudes and our desires. We know fertilized eggs grow into children that's why we kill the fertilized egg with the abortion pill or with our forceps. All that time and energy to destroy. Where is our choice of contraception? Abortion always kills a developing human life. It is not always a wise or merciful idea for that human life to come into being, or be born. Must a woman apologize for being practical? Families appreciate that.

I support abortion rights because the children need a choice. Children do not want to be born to parents who don't want them. Children , when parents believe their birth is a questionable prospect. Children don't want to be born to parents who don't want them. The woman however is, logically, the bona fide, indisputable choice maker. Pregnancy is a very big thing. In places where the woman is the property, or subject of the male, the reproductive rights are vested in him. This is how sociology operates. It is exactly what happens. It is our reality.

Except if raped, or contraception fails, or your man demands a baby, women seem able to choose not to become pregnant. Be pro-choice. Don't get pregnant. You wonder how independent, wise, progressive, fierce, modern women, who are not raped, need an abortion for birth control. That we say human life is a sacred gift, makes our responsibility to life infinitely more relevant. It is more than ensuring fertilized eggs exit the vagina alive. Reproduction is part of human life. Reproduction is not all the story. We know the ink of hurt and pain, which so faithfully chronicles human history.

Debating, the humanity of an embryo merely occupies us with vain classification. We need to ask and answer speedily and appropriately. Why is this life being grown, and who has jurisdiction over that growth? The human being, "begins at conception" concept makes for interesting distraction, but it risks reducing the human life to the rudimentary division of cells. Abortion impacts individuals, individual hopes, individual possibilities, personal pain, and individual futures. Humanity trades in futures. The decisions we make in the present.
Just because God created us from dirt, doesn't mean we're born to be dirt. We treat some people like dirt from birth.

We can diagnose death with near clinical perfection. When

humanity departs we know, or perhaps, death usually makes itself unambiguously known. We mourn, we bury, and we collect the insurance. The funeral home makes a living, and we all rest in peace. The indisputable diagnosis of human beings proves more elusive. The inability to present tangible, self-explanatory, and self-interpretive proof of the awareness from fertilized eggs, must not cause us any despair.

At any stage in the development of a human, life is present. Elizabeth the mother of John the Baptist, being six months pregnant, reports John leaped for joy in her womb, upon hearing Mary's greeting. This means John was not only alive, he was aware and capable of serious intellectual discernment. As the angel had foretold, John the Baptist was filled with the Holy Spirit from his mother's womb. Elizabeth got to see that fulfilled. This should lead us to conclude regular, unborn children do not possess such cognitive qualities at six months. For the event to be miraculous, or noteworthy it absolutely could not be the norm. We have a timeline from God himself.

When unborn human life gives rise to a conscious human being is quite another issue. Human life. When does it become a human being? As pointed out earlier, the question is academic, in this major social war. I don't think God would have been any more pleased with Herod for trying to kill Jesus in Mary's womb. Intent is the crime. Our philosophy of abortion should be a very sombre, sober one. There is nothing to rejoice about, except we spared the unborn a precariously, and perhaps thoughtlessly conceived birth.

When does a person become a person? It mostly depends on what the bigger people say. The need for willing parents is non-negotiable. Our discussions should be about child care. Care is now the verb, an action word, in benevolent attendance. Who cares for the noun? Who takes care of childcare?

According to the Law of Biogenesis, life can only come from life. In compliance with the Law of commonsense, humankind can only come from humankind. When precisely does a budding human life blossom into a young conscious human being?

Until a brain is present, we may not possibly consider the unborn to be a conscious human being. Further, just because a brain responds to stimuli, cannot confer the coveted awareness cup to the brain. We know one thing, the unborn will develop as we did. They won't nurture themselves. As we should know from adopted parents, it's the willingness, not pregnancy, which makes parents. The exact human status of the unborn becomes more or less irrelevant if they have no parents. The more viable the unborn, the more urgent the need for willing capable parents. Someone has to help fill that newborn brain.

The murder foundations of the abortion debate are unwittingly murderous in effect. From the penthouses to the slums, children know the effects of a radioactive birth. Ah! The important thing is you are alive. Ecclesiastes 9:4, "For to him that is alive there is yet hope: for a living dog is better than a dead lion. For the living know that they shall die: but the dead know not anything, neither have they any more a reward; for the memory of them is forgotten."

This begs the question? Since we all die, what's the point in living and dying a dog? Do we remember Alexander the Great's nameless foot soldier any more than him? Does this make Alexander any more alive? So what is the point? It all seems to be vanity. There is a matter of consciousness here. There is a matter of the hope of manipulating one's destiny to achieve more than even being a lion. We want some precious achievement, not even death can negate. The issue is not that we are alive; it is that we still can change our life. You have to own your life to do that. Children, unfortunately, are born our victims. They know so little about their lives they might as well be brain dead.

`They suffer a pain they can't interpret. For which social cause or ideal do they suffer heartache, trauma, and loneliness? We can ban abortion. We are comfortable spending nine months waiting for a new hapless victim.

This begs another question? What kind of psychopath does this? Who creates a little life so we can rape it in the privacy of our own home. Who insists we need a fresh supply of little boys to sexually indoctrinate at church, camp, and other safe places? We do.

We believe in development. Does laying the foundation for a house warrant an announcement of its completion? We will expect to see the foundations develop into a beautiful home. The all-important intent is there. We expect our friends to appreciate that.

Children are not self-conceived. Abortion resolves the legality of a non-binding social contract. The privilege of the State in imposing parenthood is presumptuous and oppressive. No intent, for pregnancy or motherhood by a woman, can show in their desire for an abortion. The unborn has expressed no interest in being conceived. The parties most intimately involved in the pregnancy are legal strangers to an assumed and categorically not implied multiyear family contract. The contract demands extended personal interference & interdependence. Parties extraneous to the pregnancy want to ratify this family contract, by forcing the labor of birth. A miscarriage of justice is evident as these outside parties impose the ratification. The lesser participants exercise the greatest jurisdiction. This order of legislative preeminence is consistent with totalitarian governance and not with principles of personal conscience, freedom, and self-determination. Unless the State causes pregnancy, its locus standi in the continuation or termination must ordinarily be by invitation. Invitation is by the participants, or the corresponding negative effect of personal right on the outside community. Negative effect is without a doubt not to be accepted as aversions, dislikes, discomforts, dogmas, and other preferred constructs of mere social preference. In consideration of the actual non-consensual nature of the pregnant situation, abortion instead of birth brings more expeditious relief to both parties in the said pregnancy.

Whilst fertilization is normally a basic procedure, rising a child is a personal decision of long consequence. It is insane to force the product of open legs into closed arms. We are complicating sexual activity, with parenthood, and childcare. Sex is sex. Babies cry. Sensible, reasonable people know giving birth is a lifelong decision you choose for your child. This is how you become a parent. You choose. Our morality reduces childbirth to a process akin to excretion. We eat, therefore we poop. If you have sex, then a child should pop out. All the holiness, the wisdom, the dignity, seems tragically lacking in this procedure of conception on demand.

Parenthood should be a choice, not an inevitable, irreversible consequence of sexual activity. The issue is about parenthood, not abortion. There is no debate that the union of egg and sperm gave rise to all these sorry multitudes of us. A human egg, or spermatozoa, is not a human being, although they contain all their necessary potential for giving rise to a human being. A mature female, in sync with nature, will unceremoniously discharge a unique and viable egg loaded with human life, about every 28 days. This smacks of a holocaust, period.
Sperm helps propagate human beings superbly. Alas, is a sperm a human being? Why not?

When we want a human being to maintain our legacy; we are confident our testes store at least half a human. Every sperm is unique human life. The fertilization of the sperm and egg does not create human life. It unites it. Then follows the human being. With every masturbation, wet dream, or uneventful copulation, 300 million hopeful sperm reputedly die, with their dreams unfertilized and unfulfilled. Even when conception takes place, nature luxuriates in wanton and liberal waste of active, living sperm. Usually only one in the millions of hopeful, egg-crazed zealots will inherit its "immortality."

The automation of nature we rely on to underwrite our moral decisions appears to be disrespectful to the very seeds of human life. Human life is so sacred. It is perhaps time we pass laws ensuring we don't waste human sperm and eggs. There will be some unavoidable wastage, but at least we would have tried our best. Why not marry off young women as soon as they reach puberty, so they can optimize their fertilities? Perhaps these backward societies are not so backward with their child brides. Perhaps the congressional petitions to stop child marriages from Florida to Hawaii to Alaska should cease. God could have delayed puberty to a more mature age, perhaps.

Let us speak of celibacy. How perverted it is that the staunch believers in reproduction imprison their seed. It is the abortion of the hope of human progeny. None should, with premeditation, intend to not copulate and not reproduce. As we can see, abortion is a word. What greater purpose than to fulfill Eden's mandate? Celibacy is the most decadent form of artificial birth control. Celibacy deliberately hoards and renders useless, precious human seed. Abortion as we can see begins, even before conception. To be fair to our public, those of us who scream this way or that way must prove, beyond a doubt, that which we so loudly proclaim. To promote the lack of fetal viability as a green light, for abortion is not all kosher. It is said the Hippocratic Oath binds the medical profession to help anything with a pulse; brain waves or actively dividing cells live. The zygote is uniquely human. It is not a rabbit's zygote, nor a cow's zygote.

What about a new oath? "Love your neighbor as yourself." The newborn is in the womb because this is home until birth. The job of the zygote is to grow in the womb, not prove its survival skills outside the womb. To say it is non-viable, so we can make it even less viable through abortion sounds wicked. We all, including the medical profession, are taking advantage of defenseless, growing human-life. A serious breach of our professional and social contracts. Or is it? Make a new contract. Human life existed way before Hippocrates. I honestly cannot see his namesake oath, or its interpretation, to be the basis for deciding the legal status of abortion. Children need willing parents.

Anyway, uttering that famous oath was with reverent regard for a multiplicity of pagan deities, I suppose Christians will find the oath unholy in their crusade against abortion.

Humans are brilliantly creative. Suppose a woman would enable us to dispense with the services of the womb? An artificial womb incubator, complete with piped-in hormones, motherly comforts, and heartbeat, would bring our fertilized ovum to normal term. No mother necessary. No nagging, no subterfuge. No Alimony. What a dream come true. All the newly wedded gay men, with a credit card, could now become daddies after a non-conjugal visit to the egg bank. Our favorite bikini models would not have to worry about stretch marks. Miracle indeed! Forget turning water into wine. Our miracle machine would cost only $199.95. Sorry, no CODs. Please send a check or money order. All major credit cards accepted.

Such a reality would erase the argument of viability parameters and the human womb. Sustaining the unborn outside a human womb, at any stage in its development, would be possible. I think the issue would now focus on legislation to regulate who had access to this miracle machine and a supply of eggs, or sperm. You could breed your sweatshop, or private army, with ease. It matters why children are born.

All viability grew out of non-viability, so it appears vindictive to punish the non-viable. Just because someone is small and growing, should we abort them at our discretion? To this day, we debate in ethereal terms the human status of the unborn. If you are looking forward to your baby you want the baby to become as viable as possible. If you don't want your baby, the goal is to impede the path to viability. The law should not stand in the way of either agenda.

Children need parents, or they need an abortion. If our contention remains that the fetus is a lump of meat, then that should not be too hard to appreciate. Always regard that our arms are long lumps of meat. We take care of our arms. Males. A penis and testes are just minuscule lumps of human meat. Forget the eyes, the ears. We treasure our little lumps. Females. Your beautiful breasts. Need we elaborate? Our bodily lumps all have a purpose to them. That fetal lump possesses a human destiny. This human destiny is no pipe dream. Our existence vindicates the unborn's human destiny.

These days, protection for U.S. abortions is rather grudgingly protected by law. The pro-life movement is on the attack, with a reptilian cunning: winning souls. The pro-choice regroups and reorganizes, to one day seize the initiative and abort yet another day. Others advise "Be fruitful and multiply."

Each year, millions of the unborn hunger to know: "Was our demise justifiable?" If an embryo is a human being, dare we violate his or her human rights? Females possess the inalienable right to control their bodies, including the reproductive capacities. Is this statement true, or is it over-hyped, female liberation cat litter? If the individual does not possess sovereignty over her own body, then who does? The male owner does. From the Roman republic back to the Law of Moses, fathers have been king.

Exodus 22:16, "If a man seduces a virgin who is not betrothed and lies with her, he shall give the bride price for her and make her his wife. If her father utterly refuses to give her to him, he shall pay money equal to the bride price for virgins."

Deuteronomy 22.28, "If a man meets a virgin who is not betrothed, and seizes her and lies with her, and they are found, then the man who lay with her shall give to the father of the young woman fifty shekels of silver, and she shall be his wife, because he has violated her. He may not divorce her all his days." As we can see, female virginity is indeed the ultimate thing. As for the kingdom of God, only virgins need apply. There is this very inspiring history from 1966 of Franca Viola, a young Italian woman, who defied tradition and refused to marry her male, sexually entitled abductor. It is a very unsavory tradition. Interestingly the law of Moses commands in Exodus 21:16, "And he that stealeth a man, and selleth him, or if he be found in his hand, he shall surely be put to death."

Let us digress briefly. The near-global domination of females by the males suffers from one minor, yet obvious defect. Male domination is far from being a naturally occurring reality, like female-only pregnancy, and less muscle mass. The Male, female dynamic is a socially negotiated, or socially imposed condition. If females are secondary in human status, then there can be no instance or the possibility of female usurpation of male function, power, and influence. This would be naturally impossible. For example, women don't spontaneously develop the capacity to perform eye surgery, and operate complex machinery because of education and world wars. They do, because if allowed to, they can.

The evidence of an issue is the evidence itself. If the Bible has to ask women to be obedient to their husbands, this only illustrates the lack of a naturally occurring secondary status. See Judges 4:4, "Deborah a prophetess the wife of Lapidoth she judged Israel at that time." Verse 6, continues, "and she sent and called Barak," not Obama, "the son of Abinoam." See also 2 Kings 13. King Josiah commanded his servants, "Go inquire of YHWH (the LORD) for me." So Hilkiah the priest and a few others went to Huldah the prophetess the wife of Shallum the son of Tikvah. This is a long bible study.

The fact is males do not get pregnant, not even if they want to. Motherhood is a ladies' first event. Take Mary for an example and take a cue from God. As reported, God did not swoop down on Mary, and announce "Whether you like it is irrelevant, young lady, you're having my baby, the world needs him." No, the indisputably superior God appears to have made Mary an honorable proposition. With Joseph, the fiancé, God required no consultation. It seems to have been the betrothed Mary's decision, perhaps because it was her womb, her glory.

Even if women have a right to decide if they should be pregnant, do they also have a right to destroy a pregnancy? The ability to be pregnant and being pregnant are two very distinct conditions. We may be free to exercise our choice to be pregnant, but are we free to end a pregnancy? By the practice of abortion, it appears, we find it simpler to exercise our rights of choice after the fact of pregnancy.

We parade up and down the streets, screaming we have a right to control our bodies. To exercise that right on the pliable body of a three-inch embryo, of whose human status we are unsure, appears brutal, selfish, misguided. Is it not a wide and yawning hypocrisy to aspire to speak, of women's rights, and then to disregard, with a vacuum, the unknown rights of the unborn? To be in doubt and yet to proceed is to risk destruction. To be in doubt, and to refuse to establish the fact, and still to proceed is a heinous misdeed. To know that the life being extinguished is human, and to explain it away as a personal right to self-determination, seems arrogant and egotistical and cruel. Just don't get pregnant.

The unborn puke to regard those of us who so fear the introduction of a coat hanger into our private parts, but who are hardly so careful about the penetration of an unsheathed, fertile, transient penis. To claim a personal authority, to cause the death of the unborn is proud, is callous, is megalomaniacal, and is sadistic. Clearly, some women do not scrupulously exercise their choice, to keep their independent, progressive, upwardly mobile, liberated eggs, unfertilized. The argument of their choice to terminate, in the face of available contraception, sounds like the argument of juvenile delinquents.

The need is urgent. After decades of abortion controversy, the pregnant mother is still guessing whether to keep or to kill. Think of the unborn, who is at this moment, tasting steel forceps. She deserves a straight answer. Think just this once, of Mrs. Lady, who is blessed with three ugly children. Her Intrauterine Device (IUD not IED) has just allowed success to very lucky sperm. She deserves a straight answer. We must oblige her. Why should she suffer a socially imposed grief to compound that of losing her child? You see. It is not a fetus to her. It is her baby.

Sometimes, we think only decadent divas and irreverent whores seek to dispense with the fruits of their sexual escapades. Then there are the little idiot girls, who did not listen in Biology class. We are hostile towards pregnant, unwed mothers. Well, it is stupid to find yourself pregnant out of the blues. We want to see them suffer the shame of their sin. For this cause, more than a few of us are staunchly anti-abortion. We see abortion as the easy way out. Sin without consequence. Illicit fun without divine retribution. Truly we are our views and prejudices. We err, once the issue switches from abortion to the mother's morality or better said, lack of morality. How do you punish a woman with a child? How do we compel childbirth and call it a lesson in responsibility?

Especially in what was Communist Europe, with the notable exception of what was Nicolae Ceausescu's Romania, married and unmarried alike utilized abortion. Lack of reliable access to contraception, it is explained, may have made inevitable the practice. Nicolae's Romania provides a vivid, disheartening example of children born because the State required it. Married women have abortions, and not necessarily because of "adultery". The moral issue of abortion will not instantly burn away if pre-marital sex and adultery cease. Marriage does not make childbirth automatically convenient or beneficial for the child. For the sake of love. People die every day at the hands of, or from spouse sponsored conspiracies. Don't worry, the baby will protect mom or dad from that wicked mind in the family.

Abortion always will cause the death of a child. Birth will cause the exposure of previously innocent life to our broken, compromised, unstable societies. Babies and mothers die every day. There is nothing righteous about giving birth. It may be religious, yes. Animals give birth too… routinely. The bitch, or the heifer, is in heat, and pups or calves will spring forth. They are oblivious that their offspring's destiny is the dogfight or the dinner table. Abortion is distinctly an issue of the unborn. Abortion is first a child issue, and then because of a female's proximity to the child, a women's issue.

Abortion is a personal responsibility. Abortion is about terminating the life of unborn human futures. Despite the global context of the abortion reality, we may want to accept abortion as a personal responsibility. In a manner of speaking, it hardly matters, if the law allows or disallows the procedure. We as individuals have to be certain. Is abortion murder? Is giving birth a diabolical conspiracy to torture, wound, abuse, main, and murder helpless infants? Are children the new doormats? Are children born to give shackled, socially-castrated women some measure of authority over something? Is childbirth the proverbial male domination ploy of pregnant, not hungry, high-heeled, lipsticked, and second class?

Is abortion murder? The unborn await our verdict.

SHADES AND GRADES OF DEATH.

Regard please this statistic. Remember, this is not a fact, just a statistic. According to the non-partisan, non-existent Parents for Happiness Foundation, 82% of children aged 12 to 16 surveyed in 2019, found living conditions to be adequate to comfortable. 74% complained about a lack of variety in ice cream flavors. 23.7% found their parents unreasonable. 2.5% found their parents abusive. 100% said they were not consulted about their conception or birth.

Let's not make the stats the main issue. In the United States, a small percent of the abortions performed are a reaction to rape, incest, fetal deformity (severe), and because of the mother's life is at risk. As per a USA Today May 24th 2019 article. "1% of women obtain an abortion because they became pregnant through rape, and less than 0.5% do so because of incest, according to the Guttmacher Institute. Yet the battle over exceptions for both has garnered outsized attention in the national abortion debate."

This pardonable small percent warrants as much scrutiny as the remaining ninety-seven plus percent. This is the bit we accept as murder. The number of casualties alone does not create a tragedy. If it is wrong, it is a tragedy for someone. We work to avoid tragedy. We preempt what seems inevitable. Poor planning is a tragedy. Poor execution of a good plan is also a tragedy. Murder is a tragedy. It is not who or how many got murdered.

Some pro-life think this deadly three percent or less distressing, but understandable. Those who see abortion as a fundamental right see no need for apology. Exercised once, twice or six times a right is a right. Surely, if abortion is legal, why any reason to agonize over our indulgence? The legality of sugar-loaded beverages or chocolate cake does not save us from the effects of overconsumption. Words like legal are only meaningful if they can validate themselves as beneficial and also right.

We don't have to travel very far to examine the effects of indulging in what is legal. The legality of love, marriage, cheese, politeness, alcohol, water, medicine, cigarettes, Catholicism, Islam, atheism, animism, agnosticism, Buddhism, family, Hinduism, war, or cowardice does not alter the physical properties and psychological realities of these products. Our abortion politics obsesses with spurious words, cute labels, and sacrosanct phrases. Abortion is not a debate. Abortion is death. Children deserve willing and capable parents. Society has this uncomplicated, logical reality to work with. No fidgeting, no fudgeting.

Is it legal or correct to kill a twelve or twenty-year-old individual, who was born from an incestuous relationship? Now as always, the deformed, the mentally, and the physically handicapped populate our little global village. Using gentle words and phrases will in no way alter the disadvantages or abnormalities we live with.

Can we say, "Oops, we missed these deformities in the ultrasound, twelve years ago? Let's go make it right." Any plan to relieve society of the disabled presence, we would be shout into an early ethical death. Visions of Sparta, California eugenics laws starting 1909, Hitler, and the Holocaust would quickly flash. Many would cry shame. A rain of curses would descend upon the heads of those of us callused enough to suggest the extermination of our disabled. If we think it unlawful to kill the adult disabled, why then would it be acceptable to kill the disabled unborn? This is how much difference being born makes.

We must make a complete reassessment of life choices in this new context. Interestingly, we have a choice to suffer. Imposing misery on others is not our right. Choosing to suffer is, very much, a personal freedom. Think of people who get married, especially to their high school and college sweethearts.

Some abortion laws allow for the death of the fetus if the mother's life is at stake. We also seem to agree. Mom, can terminate this baby when, at age twenty, he threatens Mom's life with a knife. Self-defense is not limited to action against rabid external parties. A simple balanced diet is self-defense. Some find it more productive to die than to battle continually chronic disease. In this life, death is unwanted, but it is a permanent companion. We destroy each other with glee. When the need for death is urgent or merciful, we stall as if comatose.

We are all pro-choice. My life or my baby's. We must choose, even if it is to not choose at all. Destruction is typical of all abortions. Babies do not die gruesomely if the mother is as we say a fornicator. Babies do not die blissfully when mom is designated married, faithful, and Protestant. It is the difference in the worldview which separates our abortions of "necessity" from our abortions of "convenience." Abortion, as we know, remains about the death of a life. All of life, answers to the question why? This is morality undefiled. We are in no way subscribing to any philosophy which puts de facto term limits on death. The morality is always in why? The same thing applies when giving life. Why?

Life is so precious. Once captured or arrested. We all want a guarantee of resuscitation from our terrorist or government captors. Furthermore, we insist on multiple, expensive surgeries so we can be kept alive just in case we have more useful information to pass on. The important thing is we are alive.

Consider Helen Keller. She was born a normal baby, but she lived to inherit early blindness, deafness, and later greatness. Miss Keller is more accomplished than many a seeing and hearing person, with access to universal education. Helen Keller is one powerful and convincing argument for not aborting the physically challenged. Miss Keller was a fine, productive writer and scholar in her time. Helen Keller and her tutor Anne Sullivan Macy are a testimony to the word commitment. There is no way around it. Children need their support group. Parents. The moral of the story is not, please have as many blind and deaf children as possible. They might just go to Harvard and be famous. To have a baby is a staggering responsibility.

To borrow a line from the movie Sea biscuit, "You don't destroy a whole life, just because it's banged up a little." Something like that. As we can see though, Helen Keller found excellent human support infrastructure. In saving the life of the mother, we abort perhaps a perfectly normal, and sometimes viable child. There is no need to interfere. Just let nature rule. Let fate decide the outcome. The reason for the abortion does not make the operation any more pleasant. It does not make the saline any less salty, or the forceps any less cold, less hard, less menacing, more comfortable, or the death any less deadly. The reason for an abortion, or the viability does not make life any less aborted. Since we are older than a fetus we cannot plead naiveté. Death decisions legitimately shadow our entire existence and earth pilgrimage.

In a world where wringing the feathered neck of a chicken is barbaric, by a cultured some, the abortion of human life should knock us senseless with grief. Whales, sharks, and goldfish have their lobbies. An enlightened West agitates for the life of the intelligent dolphin. Euthanasia for dogs, cats, snakes, and coyotes is with the greatest reluctance and care. Civilization obsesses with the wellbeing of other animal forms. With such a climate for life, it is only fitting that we have a vibrant pro-life lobby to represent the unborn.

A significant number holler "no" to abortion, regardless of the circumstance. Is it a valid conjecture, we may be more intensely concerned with aspects of sexual morality, than with abortion itself? Consider these views. The availability of abortion promotes promiscuity, adultery, and premarital sex. Abortion is that magic pill, which cures us from having to deal with the consequences of illicit sex.

Abortion, to put it in the fundamentalist context, is evil because it results from evil behavior. Abortion hides evil behavior and promotes continued evil behavior. We demand public evidence of the private indiscretions of our local leading citizens... those we don't like. We petition God. Daily we lobby Jesus. We pray an earnest prayer that all done in the dark may bulge speedily into the glory of light. Some wish to see this sinful and perverse generation reap the penalty of its way: AIDS, herpes, cervical cancer, disfigurement, scandal, unwanted pregnancy, abject poverty, and relative poverty.

We can then righteously rejoin, "I told you so. What you sow that you reap." What harvest exactly is the unborn? The evil fruit, or the innocent angelic life? Children are too precious for abortion, we believe. The unborn life is sacred. We must nurture it into life, not suction it out of life. In the next breath, we demand this sacred life be born to a man or a woman, who we swear is a companion of devils and other evil consorts. In this abortion issue, our science is flawed. In this abortion issue, our reasoning is unreasonable. In this abortion issue, our logic is illogical and our motives suspect.

We are all over abortion, in a manner loud and righteous. The mandate is to deny both birth control, and abortions to unprepared mothers, juvenile and adult delinquents, career-addicted parents, and every other group male or female who decidedly want nothing to do with the fruit of the womb. At least not presently. What is not murderous about that?

Before we deter a woman from having an abortion, is it not important we provide her child, competent parents, and a home? To stop a woman from having an abortion is not a rescue. It is a blockade. A rescue is to provide a child with a future, drenched in the sublime, honey-sweet of love. Pregnancy won't go away unless we all turn to homosexuality. Abortion will remain a legitimate concern in our lives, and the lives of the unborn. We should not compel what we can't deliver. A mother is a long-term caretaker, not an insemination device. The scales of justice favor immediate abortion over any future possibility. Maintaining the non-pregnant status quo is unequivocally the fairest, most reasonable, and just condition to choose for the pregnancy. That is how righteousness would deal with an unwanted pregnancy.

Visualize this. You don't exist. Then comes conception. An egg has been fertilized in the fallopian tubes. The lady is not yet pregnant. No implantation of the egg in the womb has yet occurred. The woman goes to her medicine cabinet and uses Plan B oral contraception. We are saying this woman has committed a moral outrage, and she is destined for hell. She has hopefully killed Hitler, and some of the politicians we know.

How is it logical to incubate sixteen or so more years of responsibility to a nonexistent child you did not intend to have? We are converting a less than ten-day-old event into lifetime decisions about family, housing, parenting, absentee fathers and mothers, taxes, insurance, hospitals and babysitters, lawyers, education, career changes, finances, and the inevitable political instability, war, death, oppression, destruction, and the baby's grandmother.

Life begins at conception. True. Your life, and the child's life, extend way beyond conception. Even people who have a career of making vain philosophy divine doctrine can understand this. The reason you must carry your conception to term is you had sex. This is all. It is okay if you destroy yourself and the baby by having an unintended baby. You see, the mother's life is inconsequential. She had sex. The price you pay for having sex is a baby. It hardly matters if the girl loses a lifelong education, which will benefit her future conceptions. That is, if she desires further conceptions. The woman does not deserve our sympathy, much less our empathy. She broke the rules and had sex. We punish. Our commitment is to continued pregnancy at any cost necessary. The unborn can die and worse, just not in the womb. We must have our exhibit.

Abortion exceptions, yes. The little shades of death cast a light over the absolute darkness we want on the abortion subject. There is never any need for abortion amen!

THE DAY GOD LEGALIZED ABORTION.

There is the human reality, and there are human rights. Human rights, women's rights, children's rights, inalienable rights, animal rights, and civil rights, and other rights. The practice of universally endowing humans, with beneficial and benign rights, is a hallmark of our late 20th-century civilization. The Universal Declaration of Human Rights came to public attention on 10th December 1948. On December 16th, 1966 the United Nations strikes again, with the International Covenant on Economic, Social, and Cultural Rights, adopted and opened for signature ratification and accession. This covenant was to come into force on January 3rd, 1976. "All peoples have the right of self-determination. By virtue of that right they freely determine their political status and freely pursue their economic, social and cultural development." This is Article one. There is a hint of human beings not being a single belief system, or cultural monolith. There is a smattering of the concept of choice on the individual and collective scales. Then there is the slightly "amusing" title of another United Nations agreement. It is called the Second Optional Protocol to the International Covenant on Civil and Political Rights, Aiming at the Abolition of the Death Penalty. This option revokes the absolute condition of death and was proclaimed December 15th, 1989, by General Assembly resolution 44/128.

The major benefit to the fetus, as an approved human being, is human beings have a variety of useful rights. This includes a right to life. We have always prudently and practically allowed for the necessary and communally beneficial termination of adult life. We still understand the practical need, on occasion, for lethal force in self-defense. We understand the need for the State's security apparatus to kill the adult life of disorderly elements, who don't roll over and beg on command.

Some wish to assure the ticklish snare of human rights does not strangle access to abortion. We prefer to classify the zygote, the embryo, and even the fetus as not a human being. We accept the baby is human, just not a human being. It stuns how little emphasis we place on the nurture of the unborn when we decree their births. There is no need to furnish God with new humans. God can make the very stones children of Abraham. Have a little faith. God knows how to reproduce. We see what God already did, with just the dust of the earth.

We undoubtedly appreciate our available right to privacy, freedom of worship, and other such staples of the enlightenment. Our gender, all aside from the internal plumbing, comes naturally manifested externally. We have it attached to or impressed on the body. We can choose to not like our gender. We cannot change the chromosomes which make us. So we are XX people and we are XY people.

Human rights seem to be a circumstance constantly in review and under construction. We can consult the historical record. It seems unseemly that one morning people awake to find they are no longer slaves. Society now believes they have an inalienable right to freedom. It is good to be free, but do they possess such a right? Women went from being disenfranchised, from the political process, to possessing a right to vote. This will be so until a female president signs a new constitutional amendment and revokes the female vote. No matter what the constitution says, children will still need dedicated parents. This is reality.

Perhaps it is useful to always link our rights to the supplier of those rights. If we have a constitutional right to vote, then that right is the property of the constitution, and that right finds expression in us. We have no personal right to vote. The constitution decides our ability to vote. We have a definite personal right to burn the offending constitution and begin our war of liberation. Constitutions change, rights accordingly amend. Rulers change, rights correspondingly, expand, or contract. With our rights in such a state of flux, marvel we should, at our brazen confidence to boast our rights as inalienable. So human beings have a right to life. So? Who cares, who gives a damn? Your honor "I have a right to have sex. I intended to have sex, not a baby."

The unborn babies have a right to life. Does the unborn have a right to life, or do we say so? Is our right to life a self-existing reality? We are alive because life found us, not because we exercised our life options. Life unaware of itself is dead to itself. What is critical is our awareness of the life consequences of a pregnancy. Not the pregnancy itself. As we all know, after an abortion, all a woman has to do is get pregnant again if she desires. The idle hypocrisy that abortions rob the earth of persons due is typically foolish and pernicious. Our philosophies should hesitate to promote bad math. We can't legislate on the contents of the womb, as if the womb has no owner. Children are an intellectual concoct of their parents. As we know, we have tragically imposed foolish ideas on others before.

This cult of conception worship is idolatry. We are worshipping the creation, not the Creator. The premeditated urging of unwanted childbirth is high- handed, barbaric, evil, wicked, sick, utterly misguided, cruel, Satanic, demonic, stupid, ridiculous, murderous. To blame forced childbirth on God epitomizes the toxic savagery of the hypocrite's creed. Man finds no virtue without choice.

Mankind has eternally debauched the young. As the saying

goes, misery loves company. Our friends share their drugs, and misery stories, but not their money with us. Our friends want us to also lose our virginity and get divorced. We do not mind that our moral rules cause others to enjoy suffering. As long as we achieve obedience to our rules and regulations, we have a success story. The important matter is we can project our power and enforce conformity at our discretion.

Unborn rights are vested in the adult domain. Mothers must invest in the birth and future of their babies. Adult considerations not, pregnancy itself decides. Is dying in childbirth a human right? Is miscarriage a human right. It is natural enough. I am not in the least way trying to trivialize, or ridicule efforts to make our lives, more righteous, less violent, less predatory, more egalitarian, and less miserable by granting ourselves rights. I note. The editing of rights is too easy. Deeds compel compliance regardless of the rights ascribed. What does an abandoned, abused child have a right too? I'm certain the children, we so eagerly save, live in another happier world.

How does your husband or the State compel you to be pregnant? Yes, remember. These have more rights over you than you have over yourself. The owner of superior power makes the rules.

The Spartans gave men who died in battle and women who died in childbirth a tombstone. These had paid the ultimate price. Above and beyond the call of duty. Since we know about the sanctity of life I ask. Does this sanctity exist only in the womb? I ask. Is life precious only from conception to birth? I ask no more. Mothers, sometimes with other children to care for, die from the pregnancy itself. This is okay and all good because it is natural. Life seems to hold the most value when it is unborn. We know this from the manner we attend to children littering the earth. Is it ethical to risk the mother's life, in childbearing, without her clear and unambiguous consent? Why are we still talking about this? 1 Samuel 4:20, "And about the time of her death the women that stood by her said unto her, Fear not; for you have borne a son. But she answered not, neither did she regard it." Genesis 35:17, "And it came to pass, when she was in hard labor that the midwife said unto her. Fear not; thou shalt have this son as well." Well, Rachel had the son, Benjamin. Childbirth, however, killed her. The sensible move seems to be a ban on pregnancy.

Sometimes, we get to enjoy the rights society confers on us. A legitimate human right must intrinsically self-perpetuate. Rights legislated, in and out of effect, tell a cautionary tale. Do we have an actual right to a lawyer?

Amazingly, we don't afford women even the basic dignity of choosing motherhood. Pregnancy is not motherhood. What if a woman believes she is unfit to be a mom? Should she go and sin some more, by giving birth against her very conscience? What if the woman is unwilling to be a mother? Would this woman qualify, as a suitable, to adopt a child? Would child services give a newborn to this woman, so she could hone her mothering skills? How is it logical that a fertilized egg has more rights than a full-grown adult? How can the future ambitions, of a fertilized egg, overrule the present-ambitions of the mother?

Childbirth is a promise of care and cooperation. You don't love your baby because you have a constitutional right to do so. Laws forcing parenthood are recipes for social disaster. I am surprised how unknowing we are of the children's plight. We talk the derogatory about ghetto and slum kids all the time. This is the information age, supposedly. You have a right to an abusive parent. You have a right to a well-run surrogate space. You have a right to two absent parents. Please sign here.

Daily we are only nine millimeters away from death, paralysis, or serious injury. The one thing we seem to own is the right to choose. We may not get what we want, but the choice is always ours. Imagine, you are born with a brain so compromised, you can hardly make choices. We can't guarantee the unborn decent parents, or refuge from deviant parents. We can't provide life guarantees, but we can demand reproduction. We are presumptuous. The unborn's contract comprises force majeure extensively and exclusively. Why do we insist unwilling women produce children? Don't we want children to have happy parents?

God, despite his ancient origins, is an active ingredient in most abortion debates. We don't have to go very far before we run into problems with God. Lawgivers have filled the heavens and the earth and the waters from the dimmest antiquity. There is absolutely no reason to refuse the precepts of Allah, as dictated to the Prophet Mohammed, as the basis for governing civil relations.

The United Nations may do well to consider a Covenant on the Universal Conversion of the Earth to one global religion. Catholicism has a great head start, as they already have Vatican City State. By 2050 this should take absolute effect. At least, we would have resolved the abortion issue with a universal directive. Thou shalt not kill. It hardly matters what we say, God says. All humans have their own God or Gods. The Christian Coalition is positive that God exists, and his command is to ban abortion. It remains that not all the human family will share this view. So what now? Suppression of dissenters has always been the preferred mechanism for achieving consensus... on social issues in committee. Isis and Boko Haran are doing nothing more than adhere to the time-honored human tradition of enforcing conformity. What exactly is wrong with asking people to dress modestly? What exactly is wrong with asking people not to steal? What exactly is wrong with banning fornication and adultery... except for the privileged?

It was the ticklish issue of interpreting God, which encouraged the dissenting Puritans to make their historic cruise in the Mayflower. Forget, they forgot the little law: thou shalt not covet or steal thy neighbor's land. God is so flexible. They all lived happily ever after. Those who emerged from behind the Communist Iron Curtain still have suppressed memories of societies dedicated to imposing the social way. If God opposes abortion or murder, or fornication or anything else accepted to be evil, I am convinced God the Father is powerful enough to enforce his law. Yet, he gives us all liberty to resist our oppressors whether they be of the legal or common sort. Thank God, we don't need anybody's permission to love him (none of this gender-neutral stuff here) with all our heart and all our soul. This is a fundamental right. It is yours truly.

We receive commands of eternal currency "Love one another. Love your unborn neighbor as yourself." Good choices do not focus on upholding the law. Good choices focus on communal benefit and light burdens. Laws reflect the negotiations of society itself. They chronicle intellectual intrigues of contemporary or past power brokers. Some societies handled the negotiations eons ago, and it is now officially closed to any major reform. We strive to survive the best way we can. We devise laws to protect the interests of the many or the few. Like our rights, what is legal or illegal is not a social absolute. Regard for the divine law is not equal. It is a grave distress that the spiritual law has the very humans who interpret it as its highest court of appeal.

Those who believe God forbids abortion will have to prove that fact, by means other than the generous quoting of Holy scripture. Many people, alas, do not believe in the Holy scriptures.

The Jesus Christ of the scriptures says, "Woe to those who are with child in those days. They shall say, blessed are those breasts that never gave suck" What else is the meaning of woe, but woe? There is a time for everything. It can never always be time to have a baby. The human environment does not allow for cruise control. This is an irreproachable natural, matter of fact. We believe. The facts remain. This abortion debate is no different. Abortion kills developing babies. Babies need adult care. We legislate between these known and irrevocable truths.

It is up to the adults, to nourish, and design the futures of their children. If someone did not want to share their DNA with me, I would not ask the supreme court or any legislature to compel them to do so.

From the killing fields of the Great Plains, Kampuchea, Vietnam, to Rwanda, to war in Syria, adults have been meticulous and careful about one thing, no child born or unborn gets destroyed. The earth's most dependent and vulnerable never shall taste or suffer adult pain, because of sectarian or national disputes. The laws of the United Nations, and our various religions, assure and ensure the outcome. Three cheers for logic. We have accomplished a tremendous responsibility to the unborn. Adults should not have children until duly licensed by the State. As we can see, reproduction is virtually a State-owned activity. So? Formalize it. Every nine months licenses would up for renewal.

Where do we derive this fantastic power to decree reproduction? Hiroshima must be bombed because it is the practical thing to do. We can sanction North Korea and Cuba into famine because it helps secure the greater good. Welfare must find its end because it encourages and engineers poor social habits. Roe v. Wade and its illegal siblings impact every minute on the life of a child. If our views on birth and abortion are wrong, the first and only victim is the innocent, defenseless unborn.

Our little human beings live or die according to our dictate. It is their life, but it is always our decision about their life. We owe the unborn a sensible and practical decision. The historical reality of human civilization is depressing. It seems rather cavalier to show our optimism, or our faith in God by having children. We assume we need to work, to feed ourselves, not to mention take our vacations. God has proven he is good at supplying low carb manna. I am wrong. Maybe he said, "By the sweat of your brow you shall eat chicken and fries." Life for a multitude of our children means squeaking through every miserable today. The reward is to inherit a vain tomorrow. Our children are born because we so desire. Please don't blame God.

A woman consults or does not consult, and she is pregnant. We expect that fertilized egg to grow confident in the hope his parents are ready to protect and serve.

Our children will invariably be born into a hostile, selfish world. One contaminated with social and ecological poisons. According to The National Center for The Victims of Crime, 1 in

5 girls and 1 in 20 boys is a victim of child sexual abuse. Who does a poor victimized child turn to? Does the child scout for a religious building? Are we creating new virgin lives to better research the perils they face? Given such a dismal global back-drop. Is it unreasonable for parents to want to be parents? Are parents planning to be parents, or are we planning childbirth? We owe our children love, not birth. Don't we know the bouncing babies need care? We created them without consultation when we were making love.

Is it not fair and fitting that we be unconditionally available, to nurture those whom we conceive? We owe our children care, not birth. We hold our children's lives in trust. They grow until the choice of their destiny is theirs. It is not so far-fetched. Life begins at contraception. It may be more pleasurable to remain unconceived. We can be born to people who grumble about making our life a special joy. For God's sake, we can spoil the kid a bit. Just a cute little. Not a big rude bit. Just a nice little sweet spoil. Life appears less miserable aborted. You can live to inherit parents who want you not, love you not, and sometimes despise you plenty. Worst of it all, you can't do a thing about it. It is not our job to judge why a woman chooses abortion. Life is dynamic. What was a wonderful idea last month, no longer is today. Times and seasons change. Adults understand that. Let's employ that sense of reason, as in being reasonable.

Children need to be born, or mankind goes extinct. Child-bearing is natural. Volcanic eruptions are natural. Hurricanes and earthquakes are natural. Disease is very much naturally available. Pain is natural. Being eaten by a tiger or a shark is nat-ural. Nudity is natural, but sport utility vehicles are not. Artifi-cial birth control, as the name reveals, is not natural. Marriage is not natural. Using toilet paper is not natural either. Death itself is natural. Embrace it.

Hopefully, we see. We can't coerce nature to be only pro-life. Nature is a prevailing condition. Nature is not a man-made decision. Life is natural, and death is natural. Nature supplies general glimpses into life. The manipulation is all ours. How we deal with life and death is our decision, naturally. To every purpose, there is a time and a season. When children are born, we deliver them into our world. They face a new set of challenges and expectations from being unborn. Birth is no arbitrary state line. We have decisions to make about the future of human life. This reality we cannot abort.

The right, more correctly, the persuasion to remain unborn is fundamental. We shouldn't impose haphazard, poorly scripted drama on the vulnerable. We have obligations to keep the unborn, unborn. Ethically, we should disturb the unborn into life, only for the prospect of future joy. We know, about receiving gifts, we don't particularly like or want.

We disturb the unborn state at our peril and the peril of the unborn. Let's try to be decent here. Forget abortion. Can we tell God we were being responsible when conceiving the precious, unique, sacred life? Once we conceive life, we owe our conception the prospect of a good life or an early death. Abortion is the antidote. Talk about bitter medicine. It may be hard for us to admit. We behaved like idiots and got pregnant. Having children, because it is natural, is selfish and narcissistic. We are celebrating our birthing milestones, using unborn folk as stepping stones. No one asked us for a miserable life. No one. We decide, and others inherit. Death is a genetic inevitability. Life is not. Choice, so far, IS the only indisputable and inalienable human right. Anyway, if we stop making kids, Jesus will come much sooner and we'll finally all be happy.

Life escapes many, judging by the number of unfertilized human eggs discarded daily. Conception is not universally available. Death is. Because we can die, it is useful to understand death. Death is sometimes a decision, not just an event. A prized modern hypocrisy is our love and sacrosanct regard for life. Even as we love, we abuse, neglect, revile, destabilize, and oppress our offspring. Everyone knows only white middle-class folks, preferably of Danish origin, make good parents. Why lobby for all these terrible other people to practice their depravity on the innocent unborn?

Euthanasia, like abortion we condemn, to be a manifestation of devil possession. See how greatly we ignore the vital life of our youths. We demand to preserve, against his will, the ebbing life tides of a vegetative grandfather. It is no secret. Nothing unknown. We lavish more attention and concern on a corpse than on a life.

We must know our symbolic gestures towards poverty alleviation, peace, freedom, and family are just that: barely symbolic. Ban welfare because of the lazy, cash trolling welfare queens. A woman is not good enough to handle a little public money, but she can hold on to a whole unique child. Hypocrisy puts stupidity in the shade... without breaking a sweat. We are speaking of other people's lives. We know how hard it is when things don't work out with our adult livelihoods.

We hold the lives of our children in trust. For all our love of life, for all of life's sublime sweetness, for all of our holy regard for the unique and essential substance of life. For all of life's heavenly origin, we create death, debt, carnage, loneliness, hunger, and misery to greet our unborn. If we want to qualify to make a case against abortion, we must of necessity guarantee our children more than our investments, or the opportunity to migrate.

An unborn child is unwanted? Let that child be gifted death. Our children deserve the opportunity to die as young as is practically possible. Having to call us mom and dad, it is a fearsome prospect. To give life is an even more momentous event. As the Christian Bible says in 2 Corinthians: 9, "Let each give as his heart stirs him to. Let him give of choice, not grudgingly, or out of necessity. For God loves a cheerful giver." So too should we give birth. Carrying an unwanted child is just another manifestation of slavery, for the mother first and the child after.

To slay an assailant, and in self-defense, is quite a weighty permanent deed. We may hardly term it illegal, immoral, or murderous. Murder and an innocent act of self-defense both result in death. Motive differentiates. To roll the two into one loaf is to feed the innocent mind, with the bread of affliction.

There is context to all our deeds and misdeeds. The important question a civilized mind asks is "Why?" This is the question we need to ask. Who cares about the law? We should condemn no one for violating bad law. A good answer to why should work every time. This is righteousness.

The English Common law works well in families too. No laundry list of dos and don'ts, just one common law tradition. The common sense of Family first. The unborn only have the adults to attend to their needs. When that basic prenatal cooperation between parents and child is fickle, the child's votes. "Abort me. Abort me early." It seems murderous of the State to kill in committee such an innocent and reasonable request.

How nicely we continue, with our propaganda that children are precious. Check the logbooks. We want a child born to perpetuate our exceptional DNA. We know from personal experience; the contemptible status of an adult who chooses child-rearing over the glory of career.

Whore is better than mom because at least, there is economic stimulation and social activity. I am not saying bad stuff about whores, by the way. How does a woman end up being backward for choosing to be a mother? Parenthood is a career, much more than a job. Yes, it's your job, when you are a full-time mom or dad. How do insults like, "Lazy, backward, privileged, rich, and well off", get associated with persons who invest a majority of their time in raising their kids? Are the kids not worth the time? We know we don't hold motherhood in any great esteem. Our abortion bans prove this. What's the big deal, it's just a baby. Baby lives begin at contraception.

Is a public apology required, for devoting more time per day with our child, than is the norm? Is the unique human life not deserving of all the time and attention we can provide? When we have limited time to devote to the newborn? Do we still think an abortion ban is socially beneficial and morally sound?

Sewers for homes, mud cakes, and garbage for breakfast, glue, alcohol and Crack, high fructose corn syrup for inspiration, prison, school, and church, for an education. You and I, we still talk about our love for life and family. Raising a family, or having a child is a personal decision. We should compel no citizen to become a parent. Children grow up to appreciate the choices made on their behalf. It is injurious to the dignity of life itself. No one should force the birth of a child. God wants our family, not our DNA. We are busy demanding other people's children be born, just when it seems we hardly enough have time for our own. The reason we typically leave our wealth, or our debts to our children, and not to the neighbors is because we know our boundaries and jurisdiction. Illogical and hypocritical that we are up inside other people's wombs, deciding for them. Babies are not appendages conceived for destruction, in or out of the womb. Especially not outside the womb.

Even politicians speak of recapturing traditional family values. We enthusiastically applaud. That moral fabric, we talk of, covers about as much as does the Emperor's new clothes. Apparently, almost since man's creation, God has not approved of our family values. Recapture traditional values and recapture sexism, racism, elitism, religious intolerance, envy, greed, cruelty, oppression, dishonesty, hypocrisy, sexual abuse, physical abuse, abandonment, loneliness, and every variety of discrimination and horrible sin. If our values are traditional, the unborn would rather take their chances with abortion. Is it too hard for God to reincarnate an aborted soul?

A number above too-many of our children now need love, family, food, and attention. It seems impossible to find men and women, and a system, willing to provide even those basic services. Incredible. We ban abortion in the face of a dearth of able adults. Who is to provide a few necessities for abandoned or orphaned kids? Remember, these abandoned children are the product of normal heterosexual intercourse, not rape, not incest.

The reality is clear. Children are not precious enough. Their unmerited plight sways us not one bit to forgo our treasured prejudices. Schools, we say, are suffering a need for qualified, dedicated teachers. Well, our children need qualified, dedicated parents. We urge parents to provide children with middle-class mansions of polished wood and stone. Heedless to our wishes, so many children waste away in shanties for the unloved. We champion the cry for adoption, instead of abortion. Before us lies a world with a backlog of applications for care and love.

Oblivious or unheeding of the backlog, we urge on the birth of another unwanted child. We speak of love for life, and then we offer blatant, hungry neglect to the little begging hands. The world is here for us to observe. Dare we pretend ignorance of the pain, the grind, the deprivation? We speak of life as if we are unaware of the stench of the yet unburied dead. We have nurtured a world with every modern convenience except love. Man has lived on earth long enough to convince us of our perennial loveless quality. To ban abortion is loveless. To promote abortion as a basic woman right is deadly foolish. No one asked any woman to have sex and get herself pregnant. If she is pregnant, we assume it was on purpose. She is an adult, and she makes big girl decisions. Now, if a woman is so irresponsible or naïve about pregnancy and has unprotected sex, does this sound like mother of the year planning? If she wants an abortion, oblige her, please. Life begins at contraception.

Being born is not science fiction. We know life's reality. We know our record. We know we fail with constitutional regularity. The formula for procreation continues. When we create a pregnancy, we owe that child our unwavering commitment to be lovingly available. A child is born and still, that child finds us unprepared. A child is born unplanned, unloved, unwanted. Bad military strategy cost lives, so does poor social strategy. Abortion saves lives. Get one today.

Nine months is a very long, long, long time to mislead an unborn someone. Where is the planned parenthood? The 'A' word: Abortion remains too terrible a deed, so we insist, let the child be. Let the children be miserable? We continue to do the 'F' word. As we are busy F wording each other's brains out, should we not spare a thought? Have we just strategized distress and inconvenience for an innocent child?

Can giving birth ever be a sin? If having sex outside of marriage is sin, how can birth outside of marriage not be a sin? We even call the poor little bastards "Illegitimate." So truly, two wrongs do not make it right. The child is newborn, and the name-calling and bullying has already started. Why would we carry a pregnancy to term, so we can torture the newborn? We know giving birth is natural, but is it always correct to do so? Marijuana is natural. Snow is natural. Heat is natural. Rattlesnakes are natural. What variety of evil is it, to command a child forced into arms? Life is natural. Death is natural. At least we escaped that terrible deed of abortion! So do we exalt?

We revel in equating birth, with a commitment to nurturing life. We continue to sponsor a myth, more imaginary than the fountain of youth. Great joy awaits the unborn. So do we affirm? That much-lauded joy somehow seems to have escaped those already born. Our overburdened shoulders groan, sore from our loads of frustrations and pains. Perhaps joy is an unborn thing. Daily, our coerced intellects allow life to equal breathing. Is it life to breathe in the despair of our polluted atmosphere? What aim, purpose or hope do we love into our children? To be is not to be.

Each blessed day we criticize fellow humans for being terrible people. Every balmy moonlit evening, we regale some acquaintance with the horror stories of our once beloved exes. Why do we insist that children are born to terrible people? We know without a doubt, the lady in our life is a dishonest bitch, and our gentleman is an irresponsible, drunk prick. Still, we want a dishonorable discharge and a baby. Where exactly does a baby logically come into this equation? The decision to conceive requires the greatest humility.

Some of us profess to treasure life. We should say human life is too precious for tacky creation. Even after birth, the appreciation for unique human life is only marginal. Too many of us are collateral damage from the immoral affairs we call nature and family. We marginalize the sanctity of life by regarding its future with scant respect. To date, it appears harmful and immoral to subject a child to any manner of frivolous conception. Do we yet believe it appropriate? Should the request for a paternity test greet our newborn? Let's not roll our eyes, please.

It is beautiful when we announce the birth of a child, "Mommy loves you, and daddy will learn too soon enough... when we can find him." Do we yet believe the vacant eyes of parents, drunk on upward social mobility, should greet the birth of a child? We usually have more important things to do than raise a baby. Do we yet believe we are pro-life? When we urge the birth of an innocent child into misery's twilight, we seek our misguided glory, as humanitarians.

We need company. We need other parents to be worse off than ourselves. The contrast is good. We appear brilliant compared to the deadbeat dad, the Crack fiend, or the semi-illiterate baby dispensers. Well, "In comparing ourselves among ourselves we are not wise." This is good Christian philosophy. It is primarily our hypocritical souls we pamper, with our vociferations against abortion, with no corresponding appeal for improved family relations. We are eager to protest an unwanted child into the world. We then abandon her to a world that wants him not. I said this on purpose. We speak of mercy and love. Our children have no one to speak to. The Jewish God YHWH desires mercy, not sacrifice. Abortion can be mercy immaculate. It is highly prudent, and correct, to abort the unborn if the timing is not right for you. It is a very simple debate. You don't teach sexual morality by forcing women to have babies.

I with you and you with me, speak of saving the children. The children hunger from being fed only the milk of our talk. We are unable or unwilling to care for those already with us. Society feels compelled to demand annually a bumper harvest of the unwanted, the undesired, the unloved, and the ill-conceived. The very fruit of our bodies is born to putrefy, and to rot away alive in our global garbage bin. Children need parents. Urgently.

Children are pro- joy. While we make mileage of the cause of the unborn, we know many continue to tread lonely, misery's highway. We would consider it folly to build a city only to abandon it. It would strike our wallets mad to build a home only to see it destroyed, without remedy or recompense. We cry when a one-dollar ice cream cone falls to waste. Please adjust for inflation. The purpose of our ice cream remains unfulfilled.

Is it reasonable, our children are born to be sighed over? Should children be born to be alone? To be wasted and destroyed, or to become a mere President of the United States? Is it not immoral, and is it not evil, to conceive a life without his permission, to inherit our human society? Jesus came so we could have life and have it more abundantly. The God who created us was not so impressed with the life we have.

When human beings come, invariably we produce death and a need for death. Is a city of more worth than a human life, or is our ice cream cone to surpass the unborn for value? "Most assuredly not," we scream. "No way," we maintain in the streets. "Absolutely not," we yell at our rallies. Every day, the lonely ranks of the food-hungry and love-starved gain new and younger recruits. An abandoned army. When it is time to contribute more tax dollars to the welfare scheme, we are quick to point out that parents are the ones responsible for their children. It then defies honesty and logic that we agitate to ensure that other people's children be born. Our money does not willingly support the concern of our talk. We are correct it is not our kid.

Why should a child be born to parents who believe they are unwilling or unable to deal with the responsibility of parenthood? We want unprepared parents to learn responsibility. They learn at the expense of children so young they can't even stutter. Why does it sound as if a new thing? The best-intentioned are incapable of providing guarantees of love and care. We, therefore, should not force the birth of the unborn. It cannot be that the purpose of childbearing is just to perpetuate a name, and human numbers, for social security, the army, and taxes. You love your baby. The child will need parents. If time seems to be a problem, abort. After love, abortion is one of the more useful substances on earth.

The unborn deserve the quietness of death to the neglect of life. The unborn deserve the secure nothingness of death, to the uncaring, painful everything of life. There is no good reason to force children upon unwilling parents. One hears of a critical lack of quality daycare. Let us be sharp with each other. It is cruelty akin to murder to urge the birth of other people's children and then complain we can't find good help. Still, we pass laws making childbirth mandatory. We should be consistent with at least our logic. We have a sound economic foundation, and we can't find good daycare? What is Mrs. Minimum Wage, and mother of two supposed to do?

We are free not to conceive. If we conceive, then just think about the child. We struggle to service our very children. We might want to stop denying others access to legal abortion. Ladies and gentlemen, we know, we don't excel in the world of paid labor, by putting in an hour of quality time. Our employers demand at least an 8-hour quantity of quality time. Truly, where do we find the extra time to meddle in other people's reproduction? We are not so generous with our money. I forgot. Not our kid, after all.

What gives us this cosmic authority to compel childbirth for others? What is so exceptional about us? We condemn others to reluctant parenthood because we believe in life? How does another woman's abortion prevent you from blissfully bringing your motherhood to full term?

The cute little maxim, "It takes a village to raise a child," is shockingly terrible in intent. As parents, it encourages us to think of ourselves as babysitters. We are society's breeding machines. It's not just in Nazi Germany that the children belong to the Fuhrer. Who are we to abort the citizen of the State, without its express consent? We don't have to raise children, we just have to give birth. The child matter will sort itself out. It always has, it always does. I am not pretending abortion does not look like simple, blatant thuggery. I am not pretending, it isn't obvious children need parents.

Let us ask ourselves why? Why did I bring this innocent life into this tempestuous world? Whose child is it? Parenthood invests in that personal bond. It has to be personal. Child-rearing requires the child to be the issue. They are the focus of attention, and the purpose for those now peripheral, but essential, concerns like the house, the job, and the meals. The reverse is often true.

The children are here because someone was pregnant. We continue with life, doing our best to avoid the little crying distractions. Abort the child. Let us make a long miserable story short. Is it too much trouble for babies to expect parental care? For much too long, managing, not raising children has been the standard.

We think it is okay to just be born. There must only be an honest commitment, to raise and nurture what we conceived. This is a choice. I have never, in my entire life, met parents so good they had the authority to decide who should have a baby. Never. Not once. Never, ever. Never. Let's have a little humility here, with this abortion business. Children need parents. End of period.

Our passions rage, our anger glows white, as we witness the slaughter of the innocent. Fury devours coherence, as the scalding lash of our anti-abortion sentiment preaches, for the survival of the unborn. When our frothing subsides, we hurry to complain about the mothers who reproduce with abandon. It is impossible to be both genuinely pro-life and genuinely pro snobbery. It upsets us, no we are indignant. Children have to grow up in the ghetto: hungry, violent, poorly mannered, and lonely. Very good observation. Not a nearly ideal environment for nurturing delicate lives. Definitely not, the environment for a romantic curbside dinner or stroll. The child is no longer a unique, sacred life. No, the child is now just one more of "these people."

Let us stray for a minute to suburbia. Do we not possess a superior work ethic? The God in who we trust does not, however, confuse our commitment to whatever, with our commitment to our children. We do not confuse even our children. If we love our children, in the fashion that we love our spouses and our lovers, there is little wonder our children remain convinced we hate them. In suburbia the lawn is green, and we wither the hearts of the children. Children are not the welfare department, or child care services. They see our middle-class facades. They see the well-stocked refrigerators, and they also see the empty families. They see the hypocrisy. They see our commitment to lies, deceit, tale-bearing, backstabbing vain glory, strife, envy, and greed.

A well-paying job and house are great. Houses and jobs do not however qualify us for the exalted profession of parent. We are righteous. We are too good to do the evil deed. "Abortion of convenience" is a procedure for prostitutes, the other man's wife, certain races, and the loose woman. Abortions are for the convenience of unborn children. You must know at least one well educated, well-paid idiot you think worthy of sterilization. What is so evil about keeping unborn children out of the evil clutches of these amoral miscreants? Amazingly, we don't even believe in contraception education either, as it only promotes sexual immorality.

As the good Christian Jesus says, "Woe to you, hypocrites." We all knew long before we had any children that people eat, drink, like company, and have various wants and needs. It is usually our decision to introduce a child into our rat race. We chose our intelligent design. We design the relationships we will have with our children. We cannot overstate the effect of the unknown and circumstance. Abortion bans frustrate the critical need to choose, for better and not for worst.

This is illogic at its most fraudulent level. Women frustrate us. Those who have had not one, but two and three, and four and more children, under their chosen, or prevailing difficult circumstances. How irresponsible and selfish we say. Then the law says, all pregnancies must end with a live birth. Abandonment and worse is sometimes a decision conceived for children. I venture to suppose the kids do not quite enjoy these character-building trials. You would almost think children are disposable fashion accessories sometimes. Born for dangling and trashing. Something like Mardi Gras baubles, but without the brief accompanying levity.

It is hateful to condemn a woman for having an abortion. She believes she won't, or can't dedicate the resources to parenthood. This sounds responsible. I think every sexually active woman should have emergency contraception if not abortion pills stashed somewhere secure. Just another necessity of life, like tampons and toothpaste. We must include time in the equation when we discuss children. We must appreciate the time our children will need from us. They need our time, as much as they need warm clothing in the cold. Are we pro-life, or are we pro-breathing? Always remember, my abortion does not interfere with your reproductive ambitions. Who volunteers to be Pro-happy baby?

Let the woman finish her schooling if she so chooses. Let her graduate to parenthood. Let her save some cash. Let her learn how to better manage her fine pair of legs. Let her learn the far-reaching implications of motherhood. The next new baby she has might enjoy all these minor improvements. We need to discuss raising babies much more than we do. Let's shower some attention on the nurture of newborn life.

Children understand that child-rearing is a full-time career. This is because they are full-time children. This is not a football game. When we produce children, we are the coach, referee, and team player. If we have no time to play, we may wish to skip the game. Children rarely take care of themselves. I accept Hercules as a baby killed those two poisonous snakes. In more recent history, though, even Jesus Christ needed parents to rush him to find sanctuary in Egypt. See the play: Herod And The Birth Of Christmas, for more details.

Our paying jobs are not the only thing requiring dedication, motivation, intelligence, and dedication. We are not breeding cattle or hens. Our aim isn't to only multiply the brood, the herd, and the flock. When we farm, we know supervision and attention is essential, if not critical for a quality product. Sometimes adjustments are a must when the droughts linger, and the waterholes and irrigations canals parch. How does a civilized mind even conceive forced parenthood?

We abuse the unborn when we compel their participation in the adult mess we call life. The abortion issue is simple. Yes, it is conceptually and sometimes physically brutal. However unsavory, it is even more brutal, more hateful, more merciless, more hypocritical, more ideologically flawed, more intimately stupid, and less loving, to condemn a child to parents who have said no. We will remove children from parental care because we think the parents unfit or abusive. Good. Nine months earlier these same parents can't have an abortion.

It is not fetal viability, which is the issue. The issue is parental viability. Let the parents decide if an investment in a child is the family business. The State should, logically, take a back seat to the citizen. Withdraw this obscene interfering hand of the State, from an intensely personal contract. The reality is this. Pregnancy is personal. We are not surrogates for the State. Until people have time to rear children, why all the arguments demanding the birth of the unborn? The State should know by now. Functioning family units benefit the commune in every way possible.

Caretakers know just how demanding and involved their profession is. The only time babies sleep is after they have first exhausted you. We all remain unqualified to demand the birth of anyone else's child. Abortion is not a contagious disease. There is no need for an abortion quarantine. Contraceptive immunization yes. Quarantine no. It is unethical, to disguise our preoccupation with sexual intercourse, with the inevitable conception of children. In every case, the child is born a victim.

With so many good religious and agnostic people on earth, it is astounding the prevalence of human misery and deprivation. It is not enough to be born. We cannot yet discover the life-nurturing medicine to administer to the millions oppressed in childhood and youth. Children are having a very tough shot at life. Abandoned, abused, cold, yelled at, not spoken to, hungry, overfed junk, raised to be oppressors, lonely, raped, ignored, sold into slavery, abandoned, whipped, starved, sold as child brides, buggered, and abandoned. Being born dead is not the worst thing, which can go wrong with a child's life. Imagine that. Today is the day. Nurture a few of those already born.

We can pretend to discuss abortion in a social vacuum. Invest love into the children already born. An abortion ban does not do this. Our loving minds daily survey the begging eyes of our abandoned charges. Still, we heap praises to ourselves. At least we did not have an abortion. We lack the honesty required to murder our unwanted children on the abortionist's rack. Oh my God, what will the neighbors say? Swaddle them instead in pink and in blue. We transport them home, to a lovely crib, all the time plotting murder. The privacy of one's home is a preferred location to accomplish a death, a slow death. We plot, we scheme, we justify. The decision is ours. The crucible belongs to the child. Alone.

Christian people should know that childbearing is obsolete. What is all this fuss over breeding dirt? The scriptures say very many things. Jesus notes, "The Spirit gives life." Not the breath gives life. The age of Adam and Eve is over. Whatever we conceive is flesh, and the flesh profits nothing. Loving our unborn neighbors begins with what futures we intend and hope for them. It's our responsibility to conceive with all available wisdom and compassion. We must conceive responsibly. It is an obligation. Abortion is part of our essential responsibility kit. Man's creation was no unfortunate accident. Strive for similar excellence. God pronounced his work very good. The hypocrisy, dripping from this abortion business, might be the actual cause of global warming.

The procedures for murdering a child at home are like those available at abortion clinics. Suction: at about three months or earlier, we withdraw the comfort and nourishment of the breast, and leave the child to die sucking at the rubber nipple. Just kidding. Dilation and evacuation: After about three months, if not earlier, every morning we open wide our arms to our children, crooning rubbish about love. We evacuate our children to their very mature minds for safekeeping. We don't have all the time in the world. Why on bloody earth do we compel and force other people to bear children? It seems so overbearing and pompous, and spiteful. There may be a little more to parenting than a solid bank account. There is a good reason our parents don't quite explain this to us.

Saline treatment: Our child is now about five or six, and she is home alone. Television entertains and educates, junk food nourishes, and a superhero comic provides the comfort of a savior. The clock warns that mom and dad are still three hours to an unhappy homecoming. A salty weeping again rolls from lonely, needing eyes. This may sound harsh. Well, best practices are all about this. The best is the best. Children must have adults with time on their hands. We are adults. We are the ones to sort our adult priorities, our workloads, our schedules, and our necessary time for self, and the delightful idiot or idiots we are in love with.

When we clamor for the life of the unborn, we remain duty-bound to designate for them the safety of our love. Babies of illegal aliens need love too. Democratic babies need love too. Communist babies need even more love. Children need relationships. Children need food and health. Children need it all. Hypocrites are we. We, adults, know we need it all. We need attention, concern, love, appreciation, applause and we especially need attention.

Invariably, we conclude that it is materially poor who should refrain from having sex. All the poor have to do is remain chaste and there won't be any of these hungry malnourished babies. If the poor would stop with procreation however, this would create quite a shortage of clients for the prison system, domestics, farm laborers, and unskilled workers. Hmm, very tough choice.

There is nothing guaranteed about the wealth you may today possess, and so we must bless our children with a more eternal source of security. Refugees can identify with this. Money goes as it is prone to do, but love remains. We speak so much about ambiance. We know there has to be more to an evening out than gourmet food and overpriced wine. We revel in the little invisible intangibles, which make the moment. The background murmurs of contentment and elegance in suspension.

Children deserve to dine on life like that. The poor are just as cavalier with the lives of their children, as are the rich, and those reaching for riches. The poor cannot logically groan about their desperate and deprived conditions, and then simultaneously find the situation to be reasonably suitable for newborn life.

For too many children, malnutrition remains a dietary staple. For an endless multitude more rich and poor, loneliness provides the only reliable source of companionship. It is as vain as it is hypocritical to wage a war to spare a child an abortion when parents commit to providing only a lean and meager joy. It is immoral to take your chances with someone else's life. When in doubt don't have children. Life begins at contraception.

Some may scoff I am promoting the maxim, "The end justifies the means." If the means are available, and the end righteous, why not? Abortion is easily not a pleasant topic or procedure. The idea of chomping on our pet dog, at Sunday barbecue, makes many sick. For most, the dog is family. Babies are just not conceived for abortion. The reluctance to have the contraception conversation is painfully counterproductive.

The commandment, as translated in most English Bibles, says "Thou shalt not kill." Which holy man from Abraham to David, to Elijah did not kill, as in stop life from breathing? Mecca was certainly not won by the popular vote. We know a cow to be more sacred than a human child. We know the earthworms to be more worthy of life than our tender human offspring. Yet still, we plead morality, and some still plead confusion. Hypocrisy. I like the Hebrew word ratsach, one meaning is to dash in pieces, according to the Strong Bible Concordance. God never said thou shalt not cause death. Levite priest slew animals every day. King Saul discredited himself for not killing the

Amalekite king Agag. Subsequently, the prophet Samuel dealt with the matter sword in hand. Moses killed the Egyptian, destroying the life of the Israelite slave. God seemed not bothered with that. Forty years later he is sending the known killer/murderer into Egypt to set his people free. Just because you cause a death, does not mean you have destroyed, or murdered life. Sometimes responsible people will have to end the life of others, and not always regrettably. We must not steal other people's lives away.

Jesus well understands this killing business, he cautions his followers, "Those who live by the sword shall die by the sword." He also warns, "Vengeance is mine, says YHWH, I will repay" Good thing too. Imagine some woman (equal rights) kills twenty- two people because they body-shamed her on social media. She invites them to a forgiveness party and poisons them. So, we find her guilty and execute her, by giving her general anesthesia, and a hefty dose of death drug cocktail. She thought it was all to remove a cancerous growth from her uterus. Nice and humane.

She dies. Where is the vengeance? Only one little supermodel body killed, for twenty-two others dead, not to mention the lives disrupted. Even if you kill her two innocent children, and her two brothers, and dig up the graves of her deceased parents, we'd have had our revenge, but the dead still would be unavenged. You hang Hitler or Saddam Hussein for crimes against humanity. Where is the vengeance for the multitudes, even though we had our revenge? Let us say you drop an atomic bomb on Hiroshima in revenge for Pearl harbor. The revenge would be disproportionate. Yes, let us leave the precision business to God.

Jesus is not shy about killing. He promises to judge and destroy his enemies. Some killings will take place. Killings in the scriptures are so prevalent I won't bother to quote. All the man says is "My kingdom is not of this earth, nor of this time else would my servants fight." Clear enough. We don't expect to see any Christian soldiers, "Killing the Gospel to everyone." Excerpt from the play: Christopher Columbus The Legal Voyage.

As Jesus told his disciples, who wanted to call a little fire down from heaven, to consume a few unbelievers, "You know not what manner of spirit you are of. For the Son of man was sent, not to destroy men's lives, but to save them." Note carefully how Jesus emphasizes our spirit, our vibes, our sense of entitlement to cause death. We can murder a dead body. Whatever is not of conscience is sin. Think. Yes, if we hate our brothers in our hearts, we are murderers. The word why is a very important component of our Christianity. "All things are lawful, all things are not expedient, neither do all things edify." We see no edification in choosing abortion as birth control. Do we see glory in forcing women to become parents? We want to cultivate a culture of loving and caring for those in need, and not just unborn babies either. A little caring, a little common sense, a little contraception, and most of our abortion needs are history.

What next? Shall we compel religious persuasions? Shall we compel marriages? Shall we decide who citizens should vote for? Why not? We think it reasonable to compel parenthood. A woman's womb is like a foreign embassy. The embassy operates in your territory. The embassy may source from the host country local services, such as security, health, electricity, water, telephone, and fire services. Although the embassy is not Sovereign territory, it is inviolate and does not belong to the host country. To further the more; the diplomats find cover in diplomatic immunity. Now, there would be little point in having an embassy, if the host nation could walk in at their whim, read correspondence, and give directives.

All these abortion bans remind me of Russian serfdom. Slavery seems more progressive, and beneficial for the oppressed. With slavery, you know what you need. Not better working conditions, but freedom… by any means necessary. In the United States, the right to bear arms is Constitutional, not to be infringed. It is a great distress to some gun owners that a ban on high capacity magazines would infringe their right to bear arms. Now I won't say much about this, as I hate to debate people with guns. Anyway... there seem to be more laws in 2020, regulating a woman and her normally non-lethal womb, than there are laws regulating firearm use.

Take, for example, the recently introduced Louisiana Hunters Protection Act. If you wish to go hunting. State law needs you to visit your local law enforcement twice. Once, the day you decide to go hunting and again not less than two weeks immediately preceding the hunt. This is to ensure equipment and shot integrity. Sometimes a gun may malfunction and cause the shooter bodily harm. You can still bear your arms proudly, you just can't hunt yet.

As Exodus 21:22 shows, God knows people can induce miscarriages. He could have spent more time lecturing the Israelites about abortion as a sin. There is no lack of discussion on mensuration, leprosy, or rape. God never had to legalize abortion, because he never criminalized it. God just assumed the Israelites would want a happy God blessed family. The job is not giving birth. The Job is family.

BABY MARIA.

Preeclampsia is the diagnosis for a woman with a twenty-two-week-old baby. The recommendation is abortion. This woman, recently married, craves just one other besides her God, her husband, and her Republican president. Her baby. Earlier in the pregnancy, an ultrasound had introduced her to her little one. "Maria dear", she had cooed to the screen, as the baby agitated. "Oops, she's annoyed," she had cautioned her doctor. "We are invading her privacy." Then she laughed, then the doctor laughed, then her husband laughed, and then it seemed like even little Maria laughed.

Now, there was a languid smog of fetid expectations. "If we don't abort Maria...I mean the fetus, I mean Maria, and I mean... if we don't abort." The doctor heaved a sigh. She was not enjoying this appointment. "Darlen, I'm sorry, but the preeclampsia leaves no easy options. The blood work is not good." The odds are stacked squarely against mom and the baby. Dad has a one hundred percent chance of survival, regardless of who lives or dies.

A syringe pumps. Fluid transparent, and cool looking, flows, and flows for a brief eternity. Her mind writhes and cries out, agonized, at her dear loss. "Maria. Maria. Maria." The next day the baby already dead, via a drug injection is ready for removal from the uterus. Baby Maria won't feel a thing.

Inside the mother's mind, little Maria swims in pain. Everything she has read or seen about abortion invades her mind. She remembers her ultrasound. Maria is alive. Her baby lips expel wave after wave of adult screams. Her baby lips throb and tremble, as she digests death, and reacts to an adult pain. She thinks to claw at her eyes, to shut them more securely, against the strange occupation of her quiet space. Alas. She pushes against the alien intrusions. For her tiny hands, the pain is too large, its extent too wide. The baby is in that uterine pain, being extinguished. It's hell. The unborn is in that abortion conflagration, being burnt into a premature extinction. All those cuddling plans gruesomely chopped up for incineration. Her baby has gone up in smoke. To the mom, Maria will never be a fetus, always her baby. Maria, her baby, sucked dry of the breath of life.

The choices in pregnancy are always simple: normally both mom and baby can survive. The mothers can die. Viable babies can be killed. Viable babies can survive. Non-viable babies can become viable. The mother and baby can both die. What factor, or factors, qualify mother or child to live? Is this a situation determined by whose rights, or whose viability, takes precedence?

Consider Mary, mother of Jesus. Even if guaranteed death at Jesus' birth, she would have died, and for her child to live. Why? Because her purpose was to bear a son and call his name Emmanuel, meaning God with us. Now, unless Maria's mother is a party to a similar contract, we consider whether she must share Mary's hypothetical end. God thought Jesus needed two live parents, for his very own miraculous son. Jesus, dying on the cross, thought his mother Mary needed an adopted son, John. This caring theme seems not accidental.

Poor child has done no wrong and never asked for conception. Is it selfish to preserve the mother's life at the child's expense? Why not see if we can give the baby to the husband after we gently place the mother in the morgue? Since it is evil to kill the unborn, how is it justifiable to kill an adult by our inaction? For some doctors, we do not ever need an abortion to deal with the mother's medical problems. This provision they claim is a sympathy backdoor to justify and legitimize abortion. Many others disagree. We are back to our abortion stalemate.

Many who have waged wars have destroyed the born and the unborn child alike. Some on purpose. We pretend at ignorance. Especially from World War one & two take notes. Let's do a casual observation of the carnage, the catastrophes, and the collateral cataclysms. Forget New World slavery, and the resultant rejection of pigmentation as an approved color. Ignore the reduction of Native Americans, to a "Good Indian is a dead Indian." Forget all these minor historical blips. Remember, only something as benign as the Great Depression, or the accidental Irish Potato Famine, or the Zimbabwean Agricultural Renaissance. No babies were harmed in the making of these laudable moments in time. An alien would be hard-pressed to believe we care about children.

This abortion debate is not taking place in a social and historical vacuum. The abortion debate sparks and burns, cognizant of the reality of the human condition. This debate affects society in so many little ways, a stern line of logic must moderate it.

Let's examine a certain ridiculous assumption. Let us suppose we bring children into the world, to cultivate relationships with them. This would demand we expect to raise and nurture children. The chosen model could be the nuclear family, the Spartan, the extended family, the Kibbutz, the single parent, the village, or some other model. Why then the great need for a mother, except perhaps to bring us to viability state?

The more we stress personal family relations as a priority, the more we get the sense of the parental clause. The more we understand that bear robbed of her cubs bond. The hen gathering her brood to herself bond, spoken of in the Gospels. It seems so personal. Parents and children go together. Ever wondered what would happen to your kids if you died? Hopefully, they won't shout for joy with even the toddler giving high fives.

This is the inspired family equation from above. Not so? We do not plan to conceive a child to be born, to live devoid of the very mother. Sometimes, the newborn can lack both mom and dad. Plus, I am sure kids love knowing their moms died during pregnancy, or in childbirth.

Abortion is nature's holy solution to a parenting crisis. Abortion is not like your typical human, always bad. Abortion is neither good nor bad. Sometimes abortion is necessary. Necessary things aren't always pleasant. You don't enjoy taking your child to the hospital for a helpful dose of cancer-treating radiation. We can stop laying legislative minefields in the path of reason. For the sake of the children. Stop making abortion as difficult as inhumanely possible. Children deserve able and willing parents. We should not legislate people into or out of existence. This is murder. Hitler would understand. I don't mean to pick on Hitler, it's just that most people know about him. The world is a mess and Hitler is dead since 1945. Okay, Hitler is alive on a farm in mississippi. We know legislation can take lives.

Life is a tragedy. Unless it is the commitment to personal relationship inspiring our pregnancies, our unborn children are born disadvantaged. A baby is hardly obliged to allow us the luxury of learning to accept its newborn presence. The economy can boom, and childcare plentiful. Children still need willing parents. Sometimes if we set a date for our conception, we believe we have planned to parent. We must differ, without even bothering to beg. We have a planned pregnancy, not a plan to parent.

We want abortion to be an expeditious business. The whole point of abortion is to not have a baby. It is hardly a war about viability. We have a global culture of infanticide to disavow rigorously, and distance from. I see this concern catered to in Roe v. Wade. Legislative roadblocks, to early abortion and societal prejudice against overt contraception availability and use, are counterproductive. Children suffer immensely because of our sex addictions.

People who have sex should expect to get pregnant or to get other people pregnant. There is nothing to surprise. Sex creates babies usually, and tingly feelings and orgasms only sometimes. This is what we hesitate to explain to our teenagers. The question is. What happens after the baby is born?

Even when we work very hard to have that sometimes-elusive pregnancy. We fail sometimes to understand baby as a daily routine, and as a recurrent responsibility. Abortion is not a pleasant concept, but there is no inherent evil in the deed itself. Who wants to be twelve years old and pregnant? This is not a hypothetical question.

With our children, we have ambitions for their futures, but not as much understanding of their present tenses. It is great to prepare a fund for the child's university education. It is lovely to provide resources for the career path we prefer them to take. This future may very well never arrive. The present begs attention. If today was the last day with the child, today should have been a great family day. The job is family. We must decide on the essential issue. "Am I ready to be a parent?" Am I happy and able to exert the intense energies? Can I make my child my priority now? Do I even want a child?

Maria was conceived to share her life with her family. Why should she be born to inherit life without her mother? We demand an end to abortion. If we agree children need families, we should not see them born for storage. We know the miserable stories of child abuse, neglect, and trauma. We know the stories. We are intimate with the sordid, heart-wrenching realities. Still, we deny a child the opportunity to remain unborn. We know this is a world where adults navigate with caution and trepidation. Even in a perfect world, children would still need willing parents.

We pretend a baby is just going to strap on her little old global positioning system and crawl her way to safety. The children of the world are by large born into military-grade pain. It is rank evil to pretend otherwise.

We are unauthorized to coerce birth. We are about family, not slave labor.

Let us go back to baby Maria. We are hardly qualified to rank her life to be of less value to her mother's. Let the mother die. The father can care for the child if she survives the incubator. Why save the mother's life? Mothers die in childbirth anyway sometimes. A lack of a mother is of no significant loss to the child. Anybody in the society can adopt the little urchin and give it three square meals or more. Here we are fortunate. The male will care for his child. For eons, the toxic radiation from the nuclear family has destroyed children, anyway. It appears, if anyone deserves to live, it would be the unborn. It was our decision or indecision as parents, which resulted in conception. The newborn once viable can survive without their biological mother.

There is wisdom from abortions executed, to save the life of the mother. This is not about if we think the abortions are right. It brings a minor fact to the operating table. Moms are critical to unborn life. A mother's life is important to the family relationship. She is the primary architect. God not only blessed us to "Be fruitful and multiply." When we multiply, we should preferably be available to nurture the results of our mathematics. As said earlier, we set the bar for child care so very low. Truly, just giving birth is not enough. It would be enough to just give birth. If the contract is to produce limbs and hands for our workforce, and gun bearers for our armies, it is okay. It is enough if we are looking for heirs to inherit our brilliant works. Just giving birth is not enough, if we are designing a family. There are fates intimately worse than abortion.

I guess we prefer the screams of toddlers instead of the ear-splitting screams of the fetus. We identify so easily with the destruction of baby life in embryonic form. I am certain we are more comfortable with the torture of delivered infants. For sure, the sexual interrogation of the young by their trusted elders is less invasive than Mifepristone and family. How can civilization not collapse? We are deleting future humans from the uterine walls. Yes, that growing human being is killed. Murder is a social construct. Kill is an unmitigated biological reality. People die. This is the bare reality. We need to increase the joy rate for the born, not only lower the death rate for the unborn.

When we exchange the life of a child for the life of a mother, should we not suspect that parents are essential? We are not even remotely understanding the circumstance of the unborn baby. To be unborn is quite a secure space. We demand that fertilized eggs, incubate for nine months, in some other people's bodies. All because of our peculiar appreciation for human life. We have a history to ask. Our great appreciation and respect for human life is a boldfaced, brazen untruth.

Even when we can't tell a female in a bikini is pregnant, we have laws telling her what to do with the pregnancy. We can't detect, with our naked eyes, the other life inside. We have pre-emptively laid down the law as to its management. We obsess with pregnancy legislation. We need to know, all this sex is not just for the pursuit of hedonism. This is good, except we are not so hands-on with child care. Unfortunately, children suffer miserably daily, because of our robust disregard for actual childcare. Once we, "Stop killing the babies" we fulfill our commitment to life. Our advertised love for life is a lie. Take a baby glimpse at the delivered records.

The very concept of abortion, to save the life of the mother, is telling. There is an essential benefit a child must derive from having his mother. Unless parents are an indispensable element in family relations, it makes no sense to abort a baby, so the mother may have life. Let nature take its course if the mother dies, the mother dies. That's the way it worked in the past. Rachel died. Jacob cried, but Benjamin lived. What we do with a child, after he is born, gives us a clue about whether we should have ever conceived.

As agonizing as it is, babies get aborted when medical necessities impose on the life of the mother. The parents supposedly sharing in love or passion conceive a child. Parents make babies, not babies' make parents. Consider that the parents already exist, forget they have two kids stashed at home. They have planned and chosen to dedicate part of their existence to love and serve a child. It defeats the entire purpose of family, for us to allow for mothers to die. That baby conception is for family, not child statistics. Laws are our feeble attempts at regulating life. Families need dedicated caretakers. As pointed out already, life is precious only when it is unborn.

The design and the intent, please recall, is a personal family relationship. It is for this purpose of family, we have coined the terms "mommy" and "daddy." We are speaking of endearment and relationship. Family is not a mechanical process of feeding and cleaning baby. The baby dies for not being the architect of the family design. Then again, if mom wishes to die, she can do so.

This is what intelligent design is about. Conception is just a little of that grand design for the child. Sometimes, we must pull out our pencil erasers, and rub out a bad plan, or a good plan even. The child is fine. We attempt to design a life for our children. The child will need a few other supplies more than a successful birth. If it takes two to conceive a child, then children need to be born to parents. We cannot start disadvantaged. Since Adam and Eve, we have found it to be no great deal for our children to have two absent parents. It is a great mystery. Why do we so urge on the birth of children?

As already pointed out, every abortion yields death. Let us be righteously considerate. With abortion, we want as many women as possible to scuttle away scot-free with murder. Time makes a definite difference in the maturity of the unborn. We know that. Every week makes it that more urgent for a baby to be desired. Earlier is better. Human life grows. It is always human life, which will need care from another human being. There is always death with abortion, but not murder. This murder charge is as real as a man is infallible. Death does not equal murder. Abortion extinguishes the hope of a human being. Life ironically extinguishes the hope of human life as well. Quite the paradox. The next time we examine the limp, or huddled body, of a battered child, it will help us understand.

For certain, we do not always have a human being in the womb. We know this because we are human beings. We know what we are not. This is although we don't know exactly when we became what we are. It is the hope of the treasure of another human being, which always inhabits the womb. In physical terms, it would be illogical to call every death of unborn human life, the killing of a human person. Personality is an apt derivative of the word person.

The hope of life is always fully human. The hope, not the actual mass of actively dividing cells, is the human being. Still, always is human life present. When a woman wants her baby, we know how tragic it is to miscarry, no matter how viable. No matter what our culture, every child inherits a life after birth. No matter what our religious beliefs, all children have parents before they are born. Parents bind the hope of the child within their adult selves. The female body, unrepentantly, nourishes the unborn. That parent, child relationship is not so automatic after birth.

We intend babies to be born to people who love them. Any interruption to that delivery of love is a human tragedy. Baby Maria already had a graduation ceremony planned. This was possible because she had loving parents who wanted to give her one.

RAPED INCUBATORS

Abortions performed because of rape, provide useful knowledge. We see there are preferred circumstances under which children are to be born. We expect a birth is to be a wonderful, albeit dangerous celebration of new life. We would suppose the intercourse leading to conception was love-filled, not hostile, and demeaning. We love life. We despise abortion. We know abortion is murder and should be illegal. We also know abortion is always wrong. We enthusiastically shower our energy, time, and finance on those who delight in having babies. Raped women we stand in sure solidarity with. We look past the rape to the growing gift of life inside. We will not make victims of both the raped lady and her growing child. A pregnancy is only nine months. Raising a child is only till about the teenage years. After that, once you raised them well, they are fine. When old enough they'll get married and leave home. The reward for doing what is right is eternal.

The unborn say very little about politics or religion. They are practical little people. We plan on their behalf. We choose, they inherit. They accept being born with whatever physical abnormality or emotional disability we gift them with. As we very well know, we don't all get our dreams. The unborn are thankful because they have life.

Death is an unfortunate physical necessity and reality. Murder is a spiritual quantity. We can't be holier than that. Jesus exposed murder as hatred. Sounds like far-fetched pacifist rubbish? Well, it was not the airliner that blew up the World Trade Center. It was hatred. When people hate you take this threat seriously.

Rape is well, rape. It seems so serenely obvious, this is not a conversation to have casually. A raped person feels violated, because it is so, intimately. We feel a sense of unease when someone leans on our car, or tugs at our sleeves. Then there is the shame. So where does this immense burden of shame come from? Society actively facilitates rapist in the nefarious work. There is the unwritten rule. The victim must prove she did not invite, or provoke, aid, abet, or facilitate, the unauthorized access of her vagina.

I'm not saying women are not very, very evil. I'm just saying some of our norms are very, very hurtful. The attendant wounds are hardly the only issue. The rapist inflicts the physical trauma and the medical compromise. Our social conditioning assures the psychological devastation. The only reasonable response to rape is a desire to kill the fucker. Why do we pretend the resultant pregnancy from a rape is a team effort? For conscience sake, we must strip away any need to feel guilt over the abortion of children conceived through rape. With rape, the abortion is now twofold. Save the mother from an unwanted pregnancy, and to save a child from a conception compromised in secular and religious law. Again, Roe v. Wade does not compel or command women raped or otherwise to have abortions.

There are prerequisites to legitimize, no abortion access. There must be no unwanted conceptions, and there must be no forced conceptions. Children are a choice, not an excretion. Banning abortion reduces childbearing to the empty rote of law.

We speak of the child in primary terms, not because the concerns of the mother are in any way secondary. We need to aggravate in our minds a respect of how weighty an act conception is. People who speak of immaculate conceptions should easily understand just how high we set the bar. Humans have a natural ability to conceive human life. Human beings have no natural authority to conceive human life. It's a privilege we impose on our children. Therefore, they are our responsibility. The results of our conception adventures tell the tale. Where is the evidence of that fabled blessing on procreation?

And Cain slew his brother Abel. And the Lord God came to Cain and asked, "Where is your brother?" "Am I my brother's keeper?" Cain replied. The contract for keeping is foremost between parents and children. Everyone else can be helpful, but the baby is not everyone else's child.

We seem certain that it is arrogant and inhumane to deprive others of life. The most common method of depriving others of life is the tradition of giving birth. Instead of abortion, we poison our children to death. Some die more quickly than others. Our philosophy on reproduction is Neanderthal and manifestly unmerciful. Human beings will continue to be born. There is no need to coerce the few dissenters into parenthood.

But there is one small problem. The sex. People have sex, yes, and that remains the problem. How can society permit you to evade your responsibility to matrimony, and decency, and morality? Let us be just and altogether merciful. Is it a fun fact, that your dad is the man who raped your mom? After choking her and a few other unmentionable things, he casually, frivolously, and vicariously impregnated her. Or perhaps your mom was so young she did not even know what rape was. Is this our notion of blessed conception? We say the Almighty ordained children only to be born within the sacred boundaries of marriage. We need our moralities to rationalize coherently.

The New World black, we have reasonably despised for their penchant to conceive outside wedlock. Don't they know the plantations shut down? Don't they understand studding service is no longer required? We force, and even encourage, the birth of children conceived from an act as heinous as rape. Woe unto us hypocrites. We bind heavy burdens to the backs of our children, before the spinal column even forms. Woe unto us hypocrites. We need space from our very children. The ones we conceived in celebrated wedlock. Yet still, we force children into the weary arms of others. Love it, we command. Woe unto us hypocrites, for we proclaim our hypocrisy to be the doctrine of God. God commands us to love, not destroy life.

What manner of joy does the knowledge, of being blessed by rape, bring to the mind of a two-year-old? What morality, and of ambition does a rapist father inspire in a fourteen-year-old heart? If rape can miraculously yield joy inordinate, we should become a nation of rapists. Watch joy be multiplied to us, as good comes from evil. Let us continue to extend love and mercy to the unborn. Let us not demand children be born into a nightmare. A nightmare that routinely encourages adults to despair, and to worse. Let the women choose. Spare them our legislative hindrances, and encumbrances.

We cannot assure our children, the economy will be stable, or the leaders of the country will be upright and honest. We can, however, assure our children, and let the facts confirm our assurances. Our children were born, because we lovingly, not grudgingly, agreed to be parents. It is no great psychological booster to find out your birth was all one big foolish mistake. A unique life, a foolish mistake? Even as marriages strain and snap, parents proclaim that the family is fine. Our children brimming with shame sometimes help perpetuate the lie. Every family has its problems, we say. When a family has stopped working together to solve difficulties, then that family has problems. Another baby rarely is the required medicine.

Our joy standards are pitiful. We have forced our minds to agree. It shows respect to God and life to give birth and feed children. We owe it to our unborn. A dignified start on their life journey. A trip for which they'll need all the positive energy they can get. Is there something wrong with this? Is it too much for a child to ask for a mere available parent? We owe the unborn humans that excellent heritage. We owe them a life, not fueled or sustained only by water, air, proteins, and various organics. On behalf of the unborn, we should summon the abortionist. I summon the pain of the trade. Let abortion right our wrongs early.

Rape is a dishonorable premise for conception. Children will continue to be born from rape, no need to compel that they are. Children will continue to be born into every disaster unimaginable. No need to force them into such. Honor God by showing the high, and careful respect, with which we conceive a human being. Show yourself prudent, faithful, and wise. Don't dump God's creation on him and expect applause. Human life is no invention of our times. Taking loving care of a human being means dedicated, attentive, skilled labor. Difficult and very difficult things will happen to our children. We need not impose it on them from birth.

OUR SYNTHETIC MORAL FABRIC.

"For your Founder is the one you are married to. YHWH (the LORD) is his name: Isaiah 54:5." It is easy to understand why societies like marriage. Whatever lovely virtue marriage symbolizes, we know its human reality. Marriage, the allegory, like human sainthood, remains a noble aspiration. Our marriages compound the inherent malignancy of each individual. Marriage is a confined contaminated space. Children therefore face the combined dysfunctional nature of both their parents. They will learn soon enough. Marriage is a social institution, as interpreted by your prevailing culture. Children are people, a flesh and blood reality. The need for abortion will not evaporate because people marry. Children need willing parents. Marriage belongs to the society who supervises and owns it. Children are looking for relationships, not institutions. There is no need to entangle an unborn emergency in the adult domain.

Abortion is mainly an issue of our responsibilities to the unborn. Our adult disorders are our specific and separate quarrel. Abortion categorically should remain liberated from, though aware of, our adult matters. Issues like marriage, or women's rights, or the lack thereof, or premarital sex, or religious restrictions, or political persuasions. In short, the issues of the unborn are uniquely and specifically confined to the unborn. Children don't want to be born to people who don't want them. If a fertilized human egg could communicate its conceptual thoughts, we'd have quarrels from the womb. Example. "Mommy I do not like daddy one bit. I prefer the other guy."

Our capacity to manufacture choice is our earliest human right. Frenchman Rene Descartes says it best. "I think; therefore, I am." Being forced to have a child cannot be best practice. I hear the anguished cries of those who demand that the abortions stop. I heed, but now I ask. "Please kind sir, why stop abortion?" We give travel advisories when a location does not seem safe. If we feel compelled to vacation in North Korea, ok. We all know someone who visited multiple times and came back unharmed. Once you behave properly, nothing will happen to you.

If gold is ever obtainable, as easily and as casually as a child, then surely we would know gold is worthless. Let us truly regard our children as peculiar treasures. Is there something irresponsible or unreasonable about such a request? The ignorant, curbside males boast of the multiplying progeny. The educated, suburbia-housed gentlemen, exalt in the well contained, double reincarnation of their middle-class genius. Yes, our children are born for our sakes. This may explain why we so casually reproach our children about all the sacrifices we made for them. Well, in this abortion issue, the unborn desire mercy, not sacrifice.

Imagine being invited, nay, persuaded to share a meal. At the end, your friend presents you with a bill. In the movie, "Guess Who's Coming to Dinner," Sidney Poitier's character says to the effect it is the sacred duty of parents to love. No strings attached, no demands for repayment. Consider our physical children never asked to be born. Consider we do not solicit any input from our offspring before we conceive them. Mr. Poitier's view appears consistent with what is legal and moral. When you conceive a life. This life must receive spectacular postnatal service. Yes, our children deserve to be born with the proverbial silver spoon in their mouths.

Jesus Christ knew his Father had his back. Consider, no child ever asked to be born to a rapist, or a fornicator, or an adulterer, or a dishonest person, or any other manner of criminal, or social low-life. We are naïve, stupid, or evil. How do we dismiss the desperate need for stability in the lives of children? Holy religion fails in appreciating, children cannot reasonably be born to evil people. Why must the righteous demand babies be born to the children of Satan or to the scion of the Jinni? We are spiritually unfit to produce children. We know ourselves to be unreasonable, self-indulgent beings. Now we know the prophet Jeremiah says the most terrible things. He seems to think the heart is deceitful above all things, and desperately wicked. Who can know it?

We are overweight and we still chug soda. We are anorexic and we still eat celery stalks. Call upon God to punish those who kill the cute, unborn children. Continue to call upon God. Additionally, please ensure that we conceive the little ones in love. Assure if it is no great hassle that the young are not born, into squalor, apathy, hate, and disenchantment, sexual abuse, slavery, rape, servitude, military service, religious and secular brainwash, torture, and lingering death. What noble foundation can we provide for our children? We are in no personal or collective situ to compel reproduction. Routinely, we lie. We cheat on our income taxes, and our spouses... no harm done. Our hobby is to be unprincipled and to call it flexibility. The baby business. This should give us a cardiac level pause.

We have such exacting moral standards. Our laws are so particular and exact. Honor is so integral to society's function. The unborn aren't people, they are pawns. Entirely too many of us are producing offspring to our condemnation. Endless human quantities are daily, being aimlessly discharged from penises, and ovaries, and hospital delivery rooms. It is not enough for a child to be. It is meaningless to congratulate ourselves that the number of abortions has fallen, when the caliber index of parents has hardly risen. The people and nations we despise are still giving birth. Don't the children deserve our care and our concern? We have to be the best we can be. Not the richest, the absolute best.

A gentleman concludes that a certain female is unfit to wear his ring. We agree. This very unfit woman, we demand that she be a mother to an unborn child. Should we not be eager to see a child aborted? Excitement should grip us, no ecstasy should strangle us. We know of the effective abortion escape. We should be thankful to see used the abortion solution. Family is a human ambition, not a self-actuating social reality. The evidence is at our homes. Children don't get to change parents, after we decide our spouses are a poor investment.

We congregate, but we do not coalesce. By our standards, a good parent is any parent who works hard, and can buy his or her children a couple nice things, or who pays the bills, or child support. Anybody who does well at school, and who the police have not yet arrested, is a good kid. Why do we deny the reality of the world we stew in? We hear often of the nice people who sacrifice for their children. Something or somebody dies when there is a sacrifice. Traditionally it means you give up something valuable to a higher power, or ideal. When we deliver a child into a present pernicious misery, and a reliable uncertainty, it is arrogant of us to think we are sacrificing our life, and ambitions for the child. When children don't have loving parents, we must see, it is the child making the sacrifice. The child lacks available parents. It is not our sacrifice; it is the child's sacrifice. We sacrifice our children and we expect them to thank us for it. Child sacrifice is at least contrary to Christianity. Jesus could have died for our sins at birth or at five, or ten. His blood was just as precious, just as sinless. No, he died as an adult making a choice, fully aware of the ramifications of his life and death.

For the sake of logic, we should make better decisions on behalf of the unborn. We have children, we don't desire. The child is the one giving up life, as we continue to live ours. It is evil that entire societies have conspired to ban contraception. We are not even discussing abortion yet. Just contraception.

Food is very legal. Think of how many go with no daily bread. Contraception has to be more than legal. To be effective, it must be socially available. Well, we can dream. Society obsesses itself with sexuality, not necessarily the well-being of children. Remember that noble Mines and Collieries Act 1842? The one which banned British boys under the age of ten from working in the underground coal mines? The Act also banned all females from working in the mines. It banned the adult women no matter how strong or healthy or willing. Why?

According to the British parliamentary record, (parliament,uk) one Earl of Devon pointed out the reason during his contribution to the debate. "In page 256 of the report the commissioners stated, That in the districts in which females are taken down into the coal mines, both sexes are employed together in precisely the same kind of labour, and work for the same number of hours; the girls and boys, and the young men and young women, and even married women and women with child, commonly working almost naked, and the men, in many mines, always working quite naked; that in the districts in which females are not allowed to descend into the pits there is a universal expression of disgust from all classes of witnesses at this practice; and that in the districts in which the practice prevails all classes of witnesses bear testimony to its demoralizing influence." Sex is a constant companion in social policy.

We are not the owners of the human offspring. We can be the caretaker, but never the owner. Society is dysfunctional because there are too many owner-parents and not enough caretakers- parents. The child has her purpose to fulfill in life. Abortion is hardly about murder. Abortion is about children who would prefer to remain unborn.

Let us revisit rape. We should not seek to escape the decision of aborting the unborn by giving birth. In the beginning and the issue will be always about the choice deemed to benefit the child. I make mine; you make yours. God will judge. Amen. When in doubt, I prefer abortion. The women are the reproductive body bag. They should decide. It is perverse to make their choice illegal. It is even more perverse to make access to their legal choice impossible.

Another "sacred" abortion allowance extends to children conceived from incestuous relations. From our discussions on rape, we may infer a similar logic applies to incest. Many acts of incest involve rape. Did Sigmund "fraudulently" assures us this claim is mostly plain old, female hysteria, and secret desire? It can be downright evil, irresponsible, and cruel to conceive.

The Royal Houses of yore intermarried. Some more intensively than others. A particular description of one Iberian Peninsula monarch used rather unflattering adjectives to describe his mental capacities, and his physical appearance. The laws of genetics appear to spare, not even royalty. Regardless, of the amount of love we shower upon a mentally disabled child, the child remains disabled. Don't just choose life, choose what kind of life? Even after our best efforts. Time and chance awaits all.

When a child is born crippled, or minus the all-essential limbs, no amount of concern, or Du Pont technology will give him human arms, or legs. Plagues of degeneration flourish, and with scant regard for encouraging and supportive parents. A child's disability remains for the child to endure. A child grows into himself. A child lives to inherit herself. We cannot hesitate to give our children the best physical and mental beginnings. As per our respect for life hubris. Respect for life does not mean being born... heedless of extenuating circumstances. We look for a motive to establish murder, except when it comes to abortion. Requesting an abortion itself is sufficient proof of murder. This is a legal doctrine which enjoys solidarity around the globe. Sounds very poorly reasoned to me.

Thanks to successful Nazi advertising, we fear the word gene. It remains our duty to provide our children with a normal genetic base. Incest many times works to create an opposite effect. When incest gives birth, it can be an ugly phenomenon, and I'm not talking about the child's face. As we regard the growing ranks of the handicapped, we may feel uneasy about this genetic line of discussion. Regard the struggles of the disabled to assert their right to life, human dignity, and independence. Dare we agree, being handicapped is no hindrance? Why do we compel our disabled to be born? Fresh additions to the disabled numbers is no salute or tribute to the grit and triumph of the afflicted. Are we saying, expose our babies like the Romans, or chuck them in the pit like the Spartan's supposedly did? No, I am saying, give us abortion access. Let us choose in our deliberate conscience. Abortion is an option, not a command.

Veterans of war cannot receive adequate and punctual medical care. Are we supposed to believe there is some great, secret, social infrastructure to aid the disabled? It will take much more than changing retarded into intellectual disability, to address the unique demands. The disabled live in a hostile, demanding, judgmental, prejudicial world. On which planet do we pretend to live? It is a hard situation to be blind or visually impaired, and even more so from conception. It is a trying situation to be quadriplegic before your very birth. A normal brain is not just another optional accessory, like a smiley face wristwatch. We love life so much. We are very concerned about the well-being of life. We will protect life from death at any cost. Abortion is murder. So we lay the little ones in their cribs. Once we deliver, the matter dies. Amen.

Jesus came and healed the sick, the lame, and the blind. What further testimony is necessary to assure us that disability is an abnormal life situation? It is no benediction. It is one more disadvantage to live with. It is horrible to so intentionally cripple the mind and body of a child, and then say, "At least she's alive." It is the wish of the unborn child to be as humanly perfect as is humanly possible. It is the least we can do. Our expansive appreciation for humanity, as an unborn life form, is legendary. We have to explain why we find abortion more inconvenient than the long term linger of torture. Our right to conceive children is our illusion. Children inherit first their parents and then their circumstances. Our right to assure, ensure, and in other ways compel childbirth is crazy. Just garden variety wacky mad.

We sit with our backsides firmly planted in a chair, our legs crossed, and our hands caressing our favorite person or glass of desired drink. Someone else has to manage the same, without the aid of these vital extremities. The life of a handicapped person remains his or hers. The handicapped are the ones left to manipulate as best as possible, a demanding and often hostile society.

Though compassion was to swamp our minds, the blind would remain blind, the lame would not walk, and the deaf oblivious to sound would remain. Even if our every indiscreet giggle were to cease, the mentally disabled would come closer, only to possessing a happier disabled brain. That no semantic can change. If on some blessed day, derision and hurtful laughter were not to answer the request for a date. Then, on that self-same day, would the deformed be more joyous, but hardly less deformed? Deformity and mental disability remain a personal heritage. Our willing hands and smiling lips can only help to make these difficulties more bearable.

Deformity and retardation remain a personal heritage. It is outside our jurisdiction to decide on anything but human perfection for the unborn. We have to accept with humility our impotence. We just don't seem so powerful after all, designing the unborn. We can't even compel a child to be male or female. A rather simple matter. Only two choices. We have no power to grant guarantees of joy to our offspring. Can't we offer an unborn child at least basic human functionality? The babies want to run, not crawl to their abortion appointments. The road to abortion needs clear, unencumbered access.

Guarantee those with those trifling physical defects, conjugal pleasures with your sons and daughters. The rest of us are busy finding fault with the major peculiarities of flat backsides, large ears, or jutting teeth, or dark skin, straight or curly hair, small eyes, and the like. Yet the other person's burdens are fine for them to bear, sometimes alone. Our hypocrisy is overwhelming.

When we discuss abortion, we can stop being so "childish"

about it all. Does our God allow us to gamble with the fate of the unborn? Is it moral to expose the unborn to anything less than paradise? Are we allowed to procreate anguish? Indeed suffering is an approved part of many religious orthodoxies. It is a choice we make for ourselves, not others. Again, legal abortion access does not compel persons to abort. It is a usurpation of all logic to call abortion murder. Murder transcends killing and death.

The gravity of being a parent should make us very circumspect about issuing our birth permits.

After God created Adam and Eve, male and female, he pronounced them, and the rest of the creation to be, of all things, very good. We should strive for a similar excellence. I do not intend these arguments as an attempt at policy. These arguments show how arrogant we are to compel individuals to give birth. This case study has billions of participants. We are so addicted to hypocrisy. We behave as if abortion is a religious, metaphysics, or academic debate. There are billions of young on this planet, and they are not being well looked after. End of story. Still, I continue.

An unborn child, listen to the ring of the classification, unborn. An unborn child, consider his or her situation, unborn. An unborn child, think of the state of his condition, unborn. An unborn child should not become born to inherit disability. An unborn child emerges from the birth canal, handicapped into our prejudice-hardened lair.

Our minds wander after our noses, as we sniff out sexual encounters, or arrangements. Bang, endless misery. Instead of washing that innocent, unborn life down the toilet, we pretend at a game called parents. Then we throw a baby shower. Miserable life. Why impose it on she who is not yet? Distasteful neglect, why are they weaned on it? Do you know a child who uses daddy's penis as a pacifier? You may know a child who gets patted on the back with the likes of a baseball bat.

Procreation. Did not the Lord command: "Be fruitful and multiply"? It is the will of the Creator, some say. We multiply the progeny with a greater haste than the desert dunes of the Sahara. What I know is we cannot deliver the earth's little faithful into the grind of poverty and adult chaos. But what do I know?

The Buddha, merciful is he, "Is man not to love life and never to destroy it?" Despite such enlightened advice, we multiply the misery and loneliness of our children. The fruit of our labor harvested and regularly dumped to bruise, scar, ferment, and decay. We gather a bumper crop of imposed uncertainty. There is infinitely more to the destruction of life than mere death. Dead people are blissfully dead. Buddhism speaks of achieving Nirvana. We live to cease to exist. We empty our life experience to become nothing. I am not enlightened enough to see the fuss with choosing death.

Christianity speaks of eternal life. We see however the careful expectation of an eternal life filled with joy, health, wealth, and pleasant company. We are not just offering eternal living. We offer a delightful and abundant retirement plan. We could live forever in hell. This is preferable to death, surely. We are alive, forever, just in hell. A rather minor inconvenience, all things considered.

The United Nations might want to pass a resolution, guaranteeing the safe access to contraception and other reproductive services during any war, unrest, or attack of terror. Just another rule of civilized combat. As said before, the world is just not morally equipped to compel childbirth.

We are not building hypersonic missiles, or squabbling in Kashmir, Crimea, West Bank, or the Korean DMZ because of abortion, or contraception disputes. When Roman Emperor Constantine said, by this sign shall you conquer, he was not leading the fight to ensure a steady supply of baby cribs and winter clothes. The crusades, the jihads, the European wars of religion, and my favorite, the British opium wars, none occurred over an abortion debate, or the need for increased rations for pregnant women and children. Responsible parents must volunteer to bring their children world peace. The need is so glaringly apparent. Abortion transcends our ideological quarrel about our rights and social preferences. Children need willing parents.

The young lives we profess so great a love for. We resign them to live lonely in the gilded tombs and ghetto cemeteries. Funeral homes. Love is on life support. To date, we despise abortion. Our morality will never permit us to destroy our children in the womb, no matter how unborn. Still, the unborn are born. Why? Onward holy soldiers, raise your righteous voices in devout chorus. In one breath, sing of murder and abortion. Blow a spirited noise, sound the panic trumpet, protest this modern abortion holocaust. In holy agitation and in blessed disgust, let us retch our insides.

Do all this and more. Ensure not one little one falls into the indifferent hands of uncaring parents, or governments. Assure the unborn, but one baby thing. Assure him he will be born to ready, willing parents. Is this a reasonable request? This is society's responsibility to its children. We seem incapable of separating the needs of the unborn from society's need to punish and humiliate the whores who bore them. Women, we insist, must learn to bear the responsibility, not for contraceptive use but motherhood. We are using the unborn, as guinea pigs, for our social experiments. Our lives squeak our screams of a need for, more lubricating with, love. We have no natural or moral authority to impose life on anyone. When people make a conscious decision to delay parenting, we could politely get out of their private space. We should just let China rule the world. The government has spoken. End of debate.

We set our equipment on automatic and spew out little baby lives. Is this an unreasonable request? Let's spare our children the ignominy of lame, brained, casual conception? We behave as if people will never reproduce, unless we do it badly. Thank God. If it were not for that quickie our mom had, we would never have been born. This preoccupation with delivering human life diminishes our understanding of raising a family. The emphasis is all about our notions of murder, and so very little about the subtleties of nourishing dependent life. This old new-age crime of conception worship blinds us. It condemns our children to a terrible, insensitive and cruel reasoning. Children want smiles, and grins, and hugs, and laughter.

Are we not sure when a human being begins? May we all know our children begin before fertilization. Is there anything wrong with a child knowing his life we desired and expected? We cannot exercise compromise on a gift so basic. Not that it will assure our children a successful and happy future. It's just the least we can do as parents. We should start with noble intentions. Is there something wrong with being noble? The preparation for the unborn, and the inherited aftermath, is the uncontaminated testimony.

As parents, we have no duty or obligation, expect to spare the unborn every complication. We play God when we decide the burden of disability or parental deprivation. It is haughty to decide anything but excellence for our fellow humans. Call it the diamond rule. It is unfair that our conceptions are born of mindless frivolity. It is not even enough to do our best. It is not enough to pledge to do our best after the fact either. This I think is morality. We share the best of ourselves.

The job is family. People don't intend to raise a family. Why do we force them to take on this most delicate responsibility? Worst of all, how do we deny a responsible family unit access to abortion? The Christian God assures that people will seek him and he won't be found! He promises to send a famine not of food and water, but of hearing the word of the Lord. What are we to say? Does God want to stop doing good? Is God fed up? Does he need a break from the humans he created? Why is he denying us his pleasant life-saving word? What if we have an innocent baby while he is on leave? I believe God when he says he does not lie. It is a lie to conceive misery and call it a blessing.

It is normally pleasing to hear talk of birth control. Thankful we may be that two children instead of five, were born into misery. This accomplishment does not allow for us to lose control and treat the two in any old manner. We demand and provide personalized service in business. There is no other way to do it these days. What is our excuse? What is our explanation? Why is personalized service not good enough for our children? Why are our expectations for the unborn, so low? To be born is not enough. Curiously enough, children need parents.

We should see two lessons from the abortions considered, for reasons of rape and incest. First, a child wants conception in an honorable and praiseworthy fashion. At least let there be lots of energetic sex, accompanied by great anticipation of the little conception of a big decision. Second, we see, we must try to allow a child his or her basic human expectation of sharing the best available genetic attributes. The unborn are incapable of making life choices. We need to make it for them.

It is hard to understand why we encourage alcoholic women to give birth. Drug addicts continue to inhale the pressure into fatherhood and motherhood. The person appreciates they don't want to be a parent. The sober and substance-free rulers say, "But no, don't you know we are anti-abortion?" Every Crack baby hungers to see his addiction end. Our underweight, nerve compromised babies are eager and keen to see their rights to an abortion serviced. We are also eager, but to save lives. Save the life of a baby from drug addicts. If the lady would like an abortion, for mercy's sake, give her a ride to the abortion clinic. Our own are on the clock. The unborn think we don't have the time to attend to the drugged life, we just rescued. They appreciate the concern but understand their realities. People are suffering and we are discussing concepts of murder, like it is an Agatha Christie novel.

When can we concede a crisis exists? That crisis isn't abortion. It is cruel to waterboard grown, hell, or paradise bent terrorist. How is it a mercy to bear babies into a torture crucible? One likely to make special forces cry. Like babies! This is the 21st century, an enlightened era. We are custodians of a civilized world. It pleases us to make an announcement. Our children are born to inherit joys unknown to their grandparents. Today, it furnishes our children that gracious privilege of being born intact, addicted to hopelessness. Hurray, three cheers for modern civilization. Will we continue to heap the weighty baggage of our parenthood on our children? Let us now hasten to the abortion table. This is the merciful course of action, not this ineffectual meddling we term a rescue.

We say, "Thou shalt not kill". Is it more righteous to maim? Is it more merciful to conspire to cripple and disfigure than to kill? Is it nobler to torture the emotion and the psyche than to kill? Is it? We have our perfect, healthy minds to destroy with drugs if we please. A drug-addicted child is born with the choice ready-made. Adults will never escape the pressure of decision.

There is wisdom to infer from the Crack baby. We must make the correct decisions for our children. When we burden our children with our wrong choices, we must hasten to arrest their development to birth. Exercise your prerogative to mercy and abort a baby today. Or we can plan better. We can exercise that sense of responsibility to life before we conceive. Life begins at contraception. Thru open, unbiased discussion we can fertilize in each other that honest appreciation for life. It is a lot more than mommy saying, "Pick up the pace." She wants to see her grandchildren before she dies.

Whine and moan, beg to defer, hem and haw. Never forget, we have faculties we can willingly abuse. Remember, our children are being born with brain facilities already misused and abused. We have our lives, however mediocre, and we persist in being alive. The unborn insist on not having to share our emotional squalor. To limit our ability to appreciate life, from even before we are born, is unfortunate. It escapes logic entirely, why we think it no significant matter, for other persons to be deaf, or blind, or crippled?

We do not achieve the empowerment of the disabled by pretending their disability is a desirable condition. We are zealous to save the unborn disabled. We refuse anyway, to provide them with the basic ease of access to our places of commerce, to our buildings of entertainment, and our places of worship. The infrastructure, or rather the lack of it, accurately reflects our mindset. Out of sight, out of mind. We do not care enough for the disabled, or disadvantaged. How willing we are to rescue a child from abortion torture. How unwilling we are to spend a few dollars to provide something as ordinary as a wheelchair ramp. There is no air-conditioning and we have a crisis.

We save, but we hardly dedicate our lives to serve those whom we save. It is unethical to lure others into present danger and compromise. Soldiers alert their fellows of the ambush. They do not casually invite others into the trap. We talk the talk. We protest the protest. We blockade the blockade. We condemn the condemn. We chant the chant. We care the care. After all of this, even blessed with two perfect legs, we refuse to walk the walk. We are eager to save every child. They run disabled, a life-marathon more demanding than our own. In our great mercy, we save our unborn children, to confront a species of prejudice unknown to us. I don't think the caretakers, despite their dedication, do jigs and dances, thanking God they have sick and disabled people to show some love.

Routinely, we insult one another in the name of the mentally disabled. "Are you retarded or what?" In our caring, we rescue the unborn to celebrate life. They celebrate life in a party, from which we politely excuse ourselves. Each year, millions of unwanted, legitimate children are born to illegitimate parents. Every year, these millions deserve an abortion service. This essential service we feel duty-bound to deny. Children are for family, not abortion. What need is there for an unborn child to choose between abortion and imminent instability? This is an unreasonable circumstance to arbitrate. Abortion I agree should be a reaction to medical necessity, not to social irresponsibility. It is an unpleasant and lethal medicine. Life begins at contraception, yes. Giving birth will never always be the best decision. Our very respect for life and the quality of life tells us so.

Please, more morning-after pills. Life begins at contraception and the morning after too. This is a very convenient time for women to exercise their human right to swallow. As recently as 1965, the US Supreme Court in Griswold v. Connecticut ruled married couples had the right to use contraception if they so wanted. This is an authentic case. The state of Connecticut had prohibited any person from using "any drug, medicinal article or instrument for the purpose of preventing contraception." The gauche manner, in which we handle contraception, betrays our cultural unease with sexual intercourse. Babies are the unwilling victims of our failed contraception policy. Our callous treatment of contraception shows the cold-heartedness we regard children with. Why would married couples need a challenge to access contraception? It may be because we want to abort the very notion of contraception. This is a case of Religion v. Reality. Contraception use, we know, does not infringe on anybody else's rights.

Sound religious doctrine should willingly direct us to uncomplicated conclusions. Children need willing, ready parents. Children conceived for neglect, and social distance suffer criminal assault. The Christian standard for murder makes it possible to murder a child by giving birth. The purposeful use of nine months to give birth, into less than presentable circumstances, shows malignant intent. It is a married murderer who views painful abortion as a convenient form of birth control. It is a married murderer who is complacent about contraception. It is a murderer who delivers children into squalor and pain, to collect more state benefits. It is a murderer who complains about his economic circumstance, but helps create a child to share it. It is a murderer who refuses to spare the unborn, the trauma and pain of a compromised brain. It is a murderer who drives drunk. It is a murderer who bans contraception. It is a murderer who drinks herself drunk while pregnant. It is a murderer who breathes second-hand smoke into baby lungs. It is a murderer who is addicted to drugs and helps a woman get pregnant. It is a murderer who says, "Ah, just abort it." It is a mass murderer who says, "Bring me your swollen tummies and a fee; it is all a lump of meat." It is a hardened, seasoned murderer, who allows the unborn to be born, still unwanted, and still unloved.

It is a murderer who tells women; they have a right to exercise control over their bodies by destroying the innocent. It is a murderer who advises "Be fruitful and multiply." We can all be murderers, whether we give birth or abort. Whatever does not come from a good conscience is sin. We know if we are being hypocritical. We know if we are being selfish. We know why we do what we do. We can judge ourselves. We endanger other people's lives by conceiving them. This is all there is to the quarrel.

The abortion or birth decision is not the prerogative of any lobby, be it pro-life, or pro-choice. Now, this is not a catch twenty-two situation, where, if you kill your unwanted baby it is murder, and if you don't kill your unwanted baby, it is still murder. There is no catch, because we have an independent decision to make regarding procreation. I am not saying women must abort. I am saying we should not prevent women from aborting. We can respect our children to be, or we can regard creating new human beings, as a trivial affair. Using pregnancy to produce an unwanted child is generously and magnificently criminal. We are collectively torturing the unborn into viability, birth, and beyond. What we bear our children into sheds unfiltered light unto the collective human soul.

The unborn have a unique civil rights proposition for parents. Give me more than your fleeting material comforts, or give me a secure death. We need to get our married acts on the road, before a cute, innocent baby can join the show. I love abortion because we have an outstanding success record with it. I am sorry abortion is so intimately female. Remember that every time the waters of the red sea depart. We spread them to pursue our sexual pleasures, and then we spread them again to destroy this growing impediment to our convenience. The baby dies. We are making it inconvenient for the child to be born. Make no mistake. It is powerfully disagreeable to the soul, to see a tiny being torn apart and savaged. The womb wasn't designed for abortions. Who wants to claim barbarity as a constitutional right? Make no mistake, it is even more upsetting to see a child force-fed the vacancy of parental care. Who wants to claim the transformation of children into human waste, as a moral requirement and an article of faith?

I have purposefully not spent time on the mechanics of abortion, medical or surgical, because this is not the point. If we make pain the barometer, then we understand why children can't be born in pain, and institutionalized into further pain. Doctors can make death very humane. Abortion makes us wonder, "Why did it have to come to all of this?" All this crushing of skulls and tearing of limbs. Is contraception unavailable? Is the woman raped and twelve years old? What the $@&k is going on here?

We claim to be a compassionate people. Compassion should impel us to spare the unborn the need for a savage death, and a painful life. Let compassion lead us to stop producing a continued need for abortion. Some business activities show success by ending. You want to stop vaccinating for polio and measles and smallpox. Abortion is one of these. Unless someone has violated them, women don't have a right to abortions. We assume the pregnancy is the woman's choice, and the result of consensual sexual activity. We would assume pregnancy is evidence she wants a baby. This is unfortunately not so.

If there was not a baby involved, our assumptions would stay stuck in the adult realm. It turns out our pregnancies affect someone else's life most intimately. Babies have a natural right to choose their life. Abortion is a deadly option we exercise on behalf of our future children. Adult women can have or not have sex. Protected or unprotected. Adult women always have the choice. Let our loving intent compel us to help make abortion obsolete. Our responsibility to abort some pregnancies is not a liberty for us to continue in irresponsible ways. "Shall we continue in sin that grace may abound?" Abortion for certain is not grace.

We should reserve abortion as a medical necessity, and not as a tool to rectify our social miscarriages. We want to have our babies and enjoy them. Even puppies want to enjoy their parents. We want to talk about baby meal recipes, and bedtime techniques, not abortion. Abortion literally kills the mood of raising and nourishing children. Like discussing clogged sewers and flatulence at dinner. Well, perhaps if we are in the sewerage business it is okay. One thing makes abortion very illegitimate. That is how unnecessary it is. Life begins at contraception.

It is to our glory to embark upon a mission to protect the life of the unborn. We can dismantle our own absurd and unloving social and sexual agendas. Courts and legislatures need not play interest group roulette with precious unborn lives. A court should not deny these innocent tots a right to death. Remember, we legislate rights. Abortion must always be freely available, so we can conveniently address the death needs of the unborn. An abortionist must always be more procurable than a politician, or a State-approved torturer. You know how a little pain drives us out of our minds. Somehow, we can't seem to empathize with the acute misery the children face.

How preoccupied we are with the mothers. We want them so desperately to stand before us shamed, pregnant, and burdened. How our joy levels soar, to see the pregnant evidences of fornication, and discreet indiscretions. How our hearts wallow in pregnant glee, to see the neighbor's daughter's career, has met with a setback. So much regard do we pay to the parents, we ignore the unborn plight. Is it holiness, which fuels many of the battles against abortion? It is naiveté, and other times boneheaded hypocrisy. We so desire to see the wayward teenager compromised. Let that baby teach her a lesson. Life is not all about high-pitched giggles and push-up bras. As soon as sexual immorality has conceived we go to any unreasonable lengths to preserve that monument to sin. Let us examine always our motives. Do we care for life? Do we care maybe more for disorder and the juice of sordid gossip? Is our concern truly morality?

We gasp more readily at the sight of our daughter's pregnancy, than the fact she is indulging in unprotected sex. We all know the words bastard and illegitimate child. What a charmingly sublime heritage and inheritance. Our vocabulary condemns us and reveals our malignant hypocrisy. Storks do not bring babies anymore. These days, highly advanced MID's (multipurpose insemination devices) perform the task.

We cannot reserve a right to conceive and then vacillate in mock anxiety with the baby product. We cannot denounce entire cultures, races, ethnicities, and income brackets as brutish, cruel, immoral, base, criminal, lazy, unholy, evil, dishonest, stupid, irrational, and lazy and then make it mandatory that these impossibly disgusting people give birth. The babies would rather die. Then there is the question of our communal habitat. As the great African American Philosopher, Tupac Shakur says in his Ghetto Gospel, "Any day they push the button..." There is an overstock of lethal weapons to irradiate all life on earth, adult, youth, toddler, newborn, and the unborn. Our legislatures yet find this to be one of the most auspicious times to discuss the sanctity of life. The people need choice.

Which one of these gun holders wants to talk of being realistic and pragmatic? Who wants to surrender their weaponry? We know it is not naïve to hope our neighbors will be honorable. They will not destroy us the moment we disarm. Why ban abortion? We have scarcely met the security needs of those already born. The unborn have a very real and practical need. Unencumbered abortion access.

There is no light, just the darkness of overlords manipulating the weak. One thing refuses compromise. Reality. The children of the world are tired of being born lost. We have no moral authority to ban abortion. We are unheeding of the unborn cries. Our anti-contraception and anti-abortion policies are baby blankets that smother our young. Peep at our home planet from outer space. Earth is all wrapped up in illogic, hypocrisy, and intolerance. A very synthetic moral fabric.

JUSTICE

It is only just. We should not punish the innocent for the guilty. They may die for the guilty, but we should not punish them. This sentiment, forged out of moral analysis, self-preservation, or logical deduction, seems the universal standard in matters of justice. Is it just, in a civilized and Christian land, to insist the unborn inherit a disadvantaged future? This because of the actions of selfish, uncaring parents? Let us eloquently babble on a bit, about justice and human rights, objectivity, reason, and especially God and morality. Is it just, to deny a responsible mother an abortion because of our definition of murder? Is it just, or responsible to punish "loose" women with a child?

When I think of abortion, I see women who know their business, and women who don't know their business. Both categories are perfect candidates for abortion. One group does not have the data on the business of raising children, and the other group knows about babies only too well. The State intervenes and dramatically inserts more instability into an already compromised situation. A woman knows when she, at least, wants to be a mom. The legislature commanding parenthood is fascinatingly obnoxious to individual freedom.

There are older women, with just one child, some with two, some with six, some with seven, some who had twelve, and I know of some who had more. Each, of these women, has a story of how the reproduction stopped. Some women with two children don't want three, or four, or any more, and it is not because they can't subsidize another child. You need not be broke to choose a small family. Some women want a large family. Six kids? Surely you must kid her. Bring it on. The abortion story dominating the reproduction discussion leaves me very unhappy. We should discuss the joys of family, not the repercussion of forced reproduction. Forced reproduction is child abuse. Hatred is murder. Torture is murder exquisitely.

People have choices to make concerning their welfare, their ambitions, their realities, and those of their children. It's not always convenient to grow a family. Some people don't want any children of their own. Why does a bedroom decision have to become a publicly debated spectacle? The availability of abortion does not force women to end pregnancies they wish to keep, except if there is a one-child policy, etc.

The unborn are yet to have their plight, of a delightfully sorry future, justly regarded. Our justice demands the unborn be born regardless of the misery index. A unique misery they alone must inherit. Is it reasonable, we boast, this spiritual impotence, to equal justice? We feign belief. How is it just to punish fornicators, by demanding they give birth? How can we create a victim in our bid to punish a criminal? It is a laughable notion to call ourselves just. Our interest is in security and justice for the unborn. Society is free to meander down justice's pathways as it is used to. There are extenuating life circumstances. We need to be mature enough to understand that.

The unborn only ask that we demonstrate some resolve. That for once we assure a quick termination to an ill-conceived plan. The unborn cannot abide to rely on our everyday notions of justice. Justice by interest group. Professional murderers have a far superior chance of remaining alive than do their victims. We are such sophisticated people. We want justice? Let us love. Is it a just deed to conceive a child frivolously?

It is standard for heterosexuals to consider themselves more righteous than the gay. Gays are useless at reproduction. Good point. Unlike heterosexuals, this community naturally produces no offspring to share our communal depravity. Now think of a gay man who invests in a surrogate to deliver him a child. We expect that gentleman had better truly want and love the child. We expect after going through all the intricate business he is not just making a political statement about gay rights, using a baby as a prop. We would find this to be very Machiavellian. Very, very unkind. It seems we want children to be born into genuine parental love and care. It appears if heterosexuals are doing the breeding, then it is open season. Anything goes because it is the natural thing. The children we sire and abandon are they an affront to God?

Is it just to tell the unborn of their legal bond to reluctant parents? Child bondage? Why is this so? Society is uncomfortable with abortion. Our justice is imperfect and glaringly so. The product of our intercourse is an emotionally distanced child. Our justice is frail and diseased when the end product of our wedded lovemaking is an unloved, unwanted child. Our justice is unsound, when it assures shame, as the first inheritance for our offspring. Our concerns of justice have sands of hypocrisy for foundations. For the unborn, let there be justice, let there be abortion.

LIFE STILL BEGINS AT CONTRACEPTION.

Society pretends it is newborn. However elegant we make it, barbarity defines human civilization. It is our constant and closest companion. The world is obvious in its failings. The contempt we stockpile, for everyone else, shows only a chosen few are living up to the required human potential. We criticize people for reproducing, and we reprove the same for using contraception. According to some moral conventions, artificial contraception is inappropriate technology even for the married. We want moral rules to govern our societies. Good. Children, oblivious to the complexity of our rule-making processes, want good parental care. We have an adult word called love to describe that need.

According to a majority holy opinion, the contraception needs of the unmarried are artificial. The pregnancies, however, of the unmarried are very real. A child is a child. We cannot pretend a lack of interest in the contraception needs of the unborn. Can we produce Holy life in the unsanitary, unholy conditions? It should alarm us when we urge on parenthood, regardless of the peril the children may be born into.

After having provided half of the genomes needed for conception, where is the fifty-fifty veto of the male? I do not get a refund for my sperm if an abortion occurs. I know of no progressive laws, except for child support, involving men in childcare. I lie. There is paternal leave. Good stuff. Do men have a right of injunction to recall their sperm if they, or the female, decide on an abortion? Do men get to sue for compensation for being deprived of an offspring? You just aborted my darling baby. Talk about a diplomatically compromised male. The legal tenure of abortion as an exclusively female right fails all muster.

Abortion is hardly the poster tragedy for babies. It is sexism. We all get born into its quicksand. A woman's traditional job is to nurture the next generation of oppressors. Our communal ownership of the female form and sexuality, buttresses our attitudes on contraception and childcare. The Books of Moses, Deuteronomy, Leviticus, etc. shows how vested a woman's person is in the male, her father or husband. Even saying whose widow you are is beneficial. Especially conspicuous is Leviticus 12: 1-6, where the days of uncleanness double after giving birth to a female child. Leviticus 27, speaks of fifty shekels for a man and thirty shekels for a woman as the price for a vow. The discrepancy is obvious. Perhaps it was back pay to women for having a nine-month pregnancy, not to mention danger pay for childbirth. By the way, this makes sense, providing God is the male and we are the woman.

With interpretation lies the danger. We are assured all have sinned and fallen short of the glory of God. If we conclude women are not entirely 100% equally human to males then what are they? We could reasonably expect that a woman without a man to vouch for her would find herself socially compromised. Children born to these women would reasonably inherit the status conferred by their mother, or that demanded by the father. Now a baby is born hoping that society places a priority and premium on the reproductive health services of their mothers. Because of a mother's inferior status, it stands to reason that the babies would be normally delivered into healthcare and social mediocrity.

How we cater to the social hierarchy is evident. The president does not sit on the plastic chair in the back of the room.

Unless it is for a good photo op. True. If the society devalues its women, we can anticipate a corresponding reflection of that premise in the services and opportunities they enjoy. Malcolm X said the most disrespected person in America is a black woman. Imagine half that disrespect came from black males. During the time of Jean-Claude Duvalier. One writer theorized that the most oppressed person on earth was black, female, and Haitian. He also said, "Being oppressed does not mean you are nice."

So babies are born daily, to share their mothers' sometimes precarious survival index. Our program to protect baby lives is undermined and sabotaged by our cultural proclivity for sexism.

The New Testament in its famous, "Let your women keep silent in the church" resonates well with its scriptural foundations. Our girls need to think of reproductive responsibility. It is their right. They are the ones who carry the babies. They need to know early. They have critical life decisions to make for themselves and their children. Women alone carry the babies. All our origin is eventually a woman heavy event. People are people, not incubators. We know society preaches in all its colors, cultures, and doctrines, overwhelmingly an inferior female. Girls learn this truth so early in life, puberty is still just a bloody dream. We do not shower investments on what we hold in low esteem. The sanctity of life story is a privileged hoax.

Using contraception helps equalize the gender equation, but not as much as we imagine. In racist terms, black men, or males of any other secondary ethnicity are not second class because they get pregnant. A Gyspy man is first a Gypsy and then a man. We can oppress and hold in contempt whomsoever we conquer. Wealth may buy more social access, but hardly more substantive change to the discriminatory bedrock. Contraception is curiously for the benefit of our children. Those born and unborn. We can attest, thru contraception use, we value and respect the life of others. Contraception promotes life by prudent and intelligent decision. Children are born into toxic sociology, and they must be born with care.

Jesus preaches there is neither male, nor female, Jew, or Gentile, slave, or free. Our life defined by our common humanity, infuses us with a common spirit. We can all identify with wanting what's best for ourselves. While a woman gives birth in pain, we do not expect that the child is born for pain. We intend all that morning sickness and travail is for future joy, not only for a present birth. This notion of choice, and of choosing what is good, permeates the scripture. God urges us to choose life. Choose. Life to God is beyond our ability to breathe. We seem not to care how the children are born. We just need to see them be born alive. Our fascination with the miracle of life compels our obligation to nurture. Our moral duty to love one another should fascinate us even more. We have made the giving of birth to equal love. This is not the evidence before us, not in our near or ancient history.

Imposing our will on others is a chronic human defect. The world supports the caste system, and I suppose we always will. Is it fair to become born, to enjoy gender, or ethnic, or class-based slavery or humiliation? Which unborn life has ever commissioned himself or herself into oppression, chaos, captivity, depression, and abuse? Which one of these conceived human beings hooked up to their mother's uterus, so they could get a head start researching drug abuse? Is it moral that we compel a child to be born unwanted? Are there methods less injurious than pregnancy to help keep females appropriately sedated and culturally compliant?

Are there no other means to achieve dogma domination without the use of the unborn? Is it moral for a child to be a tool of social control? All morality must begin with the fate and circumstance of the unborn. It is a reverse process. We design an entire human life, for a prosperous future, before the future begins. That's the concept of life. This is not about making dates for a conception. This is not about trimesters or viability. This is about trading in futures. It's about welcoming the possibilities, for better and not for worse. It is about being committed to the long term commitment of being a parent.

The contraception needs of the unborn, invariably get tangled with adult moral preferences. Just in passing. Does a religious or faith-based business have a constitutional right to withhold taxes? It is clear the government openly and unambiguously engages in activities unsavory even to the worldly among us.

We confuse morality and love with a list of deeds. Love is not, by any means, marriage, or childbirth. It says God is love. These nuptial and birthing requirements, which so form a basis for our secular and Christian ethic, have proven themselves oppressive, archaic, and irrelevant. Make no mistake, marriage can do nothing, and has done nothing to dignify sex. In the human context, marriage will benefit your children with as much stability and security as will the dog in the kennel outside... maybe less. If we do your homework honestly, we must see the intrinsic failure of marriage. It is still two bad people having sex. Okay, it is one terrible person masturbating. Holy matrimony does not make anyone holy, unless the person you marry is holy.

Religions typically accept people to be flawed. Hence the therapeutic, and redemptive mandates of religion. We see that it is the integrity and stability the people bring to the union which makes marriage a blessing. It is not the institution itself. Even more so, childbirth will never automatically yield even the barest of dividend to the unborn. But who cares? We are happy we are alive.

The Bible says the heart of man is deceitful and desperately wicked. If a human being requests an abortion, it staggers logic we should deny. Who cares what fraudulent promise we make to each other at our weddings? Our God or Gods have already said we are less than kosher. A law has to be self-fulfilling in its positive effects. If marriage is good there would never be a bad one, and sinful people would not get married. This is another book.

Humanity has failed at family long enough for us to be sure we compromise ourselves as parents. It is immoral to coerce and compel people into parenthood. It probably is beneficial for children to find themselves eagerly expected. Some parents are very practical. They know the timing of their current pregnancy is not optimal. Blessed is the woman if she has a supportive mate.

Think of the sexually abused children, whose abusers have quaint titles, like mom and dad. How affectionate we are, in our deceptions. The trials and tortures we disavow for ourselves as adults, we accept as normal for our children. Misery is just another rite of passage for the little unborn ones too. Life is no bed of roses. What did the unborn realistically expect to inherit? How classically Stoic. Everyone typically adopts, some bodily discipline to substitute, for the moral vacancy of our minds. Give birth. We do well. Protest contraception. We do even better. Sexual morality, as defined by our religious executives, might endow us, with as much spiritual advantage, as winning first prize in a sporting event.

Incredibly, the marriages of heretics, infidels, unbelievers, and atheists can all be valid. These men and women do not believe in the truth, how can their unions be holy? Terrorists get married too. An intercourse till you bust program yields no moralizing returns either. The porn people of California know you need regular transparent testing. Their lives depend on it. If, "life is not about food and drink" it is not about sexual intercourse. Yes, we forget. Love one another. Love is genuine, love is unselfish, and love kills when necessary.

It is plain, unloving irresponsibility, to leave behind young lives like leaf litter wherever the sperm falls. We have to be vigilant. We endanger unborn life with our sexual preferences, whether they be socially acceptable, or socially deviant. Children just ask for committed parental care. What we need to ask is, "Who will take care of this baby after she is born"? Is abortion murder? That is not the question of relevance. Is abortion murder?" This is a question about our definition of murder? This is a question about a word, and what meaning we attach to it, in which circumstance. Why are we debating words, when there are legitimate baby issues to deal with? We have to choose between life and death. We wake up and find ourselves pregnant, what choice do we make?

Regardless of our religious beliefs, or cultural persuasions, people who are born will always need their question answered. "Who will take care of me?" If we meet someone drowning is our first question going to be "Hey is it legal to fish you out?" In some jurisdictions, it would be prudent to ask. Abortion and contraception are about the unborn, not about us. There is therefore no need to speak of sexual immorality. The sexually immoral are being immoral. The unborn deserve protection from these immoral people. It is that simple. Morality is consistent with its smallest denominator. You should not deliver friends into squalor and oppression; spiritual, or otherwise. To create another human being is no giggling matter. Ethically, it is above all our pay grades. Contraception hints we may be a little sane and humane.

Why all these battles for justice, equality, especially freedom? We have fought how many wars with the innocent young, as direct targets and as approved collateral damage. We call men barbaric and war criminals, for ill-treating grown men. The hands of the prisoners, before they were thrown up in surrender, once held lethal weapons. We sympathize yet with their cruel plight. We are happy when Rambo frees the imprisoned, but not the Muslim Rohingya babies.

What is our concern for the unborn? Conceived for similar hells, we urge on yet their births. The unborn are routinely born, condemned into conditions, which make seasoned warriors recant manhood. Why is it only permissible to make our offspring suffer after they are born? This is our record. We condemn uninformed and unconceived people to life in prison. These people were not offered the least opportunity to appeal our decision.

Our reasoning is fraudulent and hypocritical. There are disabled children, chained to beds, and table legs, as we discuss viability. Babes are gasping for another hit of Crack and Methamphetamine, or something more elegantly prescribed. Even as we speak of morality and contraception. Let a pure conscience be our guide in navigating these moral terrains. The moral high ground is not always obvious. The high ground we usually see is just the accumulated detritus of successive generations, piled miles high. Not Mount Zion.

Various cultures approve death, whippings, and ostracism for sexual misdeeds. How, how, how do these miscreants qualify as noble parents? When a woman is stoned to death for adultery, did the Bible, for example, command she first deliver the possible bastard seed within her? No, it does not. Innocent human life, possibly, stoned to death.

Contrary to ancient and to modern hypocrisy. Marriage would have had to be also about sex, not only about having children. We are only having kids because we first had an interest in sex. The brothels prove that eternal fact. Why is it a sin to use contraception? The unborn are not asking what makes up our religious beliefs. The unborn are asking, "Does this rule make sense? Who will take care of me?" Well, you have faith? Have it to yourself.

It is easy to understanding unrestricted breeding for generating new slaves, or soldiers, mothers, and consumers, but not for building a family. Note, slave breeders try to be selective about their stock.

We are nervous about human sexuality. Prudishness masquerades for fidelity and chastity. Marriage is anxiously recommended. It provides a lawful setting, where females especially can sexually waste away... and nice men too. Nature evidences it may not be sinful to be married, and not produce a child. Remember, we hold what is natural in high regard. Some women are barren. Before evolution. Females, always conniving, designed themselves to reach menopause. A woman of fifty-five can get married; it is unlikely that this union will produce a new herd of kids. It will probably enough produce more than an orgasm or two. Why don't we require women past fertility age, refrain from marriage and sexual intercourse? Are barren women to refrain from sexual intercourse? Ask Sarah, ask Rebecca, ask Rachel, ask Samson's mom, ask Elizabeth, ask Samuel's mom. Few things are as misused as sex. The unmarried abuse it, and the married scantly use it. At least with each other. Just guessing.

In this sex issue, what seems to rivet our attention is not our God-given ability, for endless coital oneness. The two shall be one flesh. This is mandatory. This produces children. We focus with a pregnant zeal on his blessing, "Be fruitful and multiply, fill the earth and subdue it." Since the wicked, the profligate, and the righteous and pious can procreate with equal ease, what is the special blessing in having children, or sex?

The most demented amongst us can be parents, and we say to that "Hurray!" "It is not good for the man to be alone," so said God. And the fun started. This delightful blessing to reproduce, God conferred initially on Adam and Eve, living in the lap of nature's luxury. They must have had a mandate to single-handedly produce five billion children. Notice God bestowed the blessing to be fruitful and multiply, on the couple, before their sin. It would have been irresponsible of God, to bless the sinful and rebellious Adam and Eve.

This is just to note, God had Adam and Eve thinking about sex before the proverbial fall of man. He said and the two shall be one flesh.

Be fruitful and multiply. What blessing did we just conceive that life into? We know every way of man is right in his own eyes. When a human being hesitates to reproduce, we should stand down.

Contrary to a popular contention, there are maybe not too many people on earth. There are too many oppressed, unhappy, dehumanized people. There are too many materially needy people. There are too many emotionally compromised people. We cannot choose to multiply children into an evil world and call it a blessing. Who asked you? Is this present world the environment God chose for families to grow in?

We must not make excuses for God. God must make sense,

or God is not God. We may wish to take the blame for God, or admit we don't understand what God is saying. The requirement remains, the God must add up. As previously mentioned. God's who publish should expect public inquiry into their erstwhile policies. The policy banning contraception does not add up. The ban subtracts greatly, from our credibility, as custodians of the Word.

It is more presumptuous an act, to conceive a life, than it is to abort a life. Remember that. There are multiple millions of children warehoused, awaiting love, and the comfort. There is a living miserable backlog of emotionally emaciated young lives. Ours is the duty to help clear it. The administration of reproduction is a personal responsibility. Social intervention is a prerogative of collective power. Mobilization of that communal right to regulate behavior should be with the greatest restraint, humility, and discretion.

Jesus Christ warns it is not always convenient to be a child, in the spirit or the flesh. Jesus speaks of trying times. He says: "Woe unto them that are with child, in those days." So much for unbridled procreation. Now, if we adopt a baby, she will suffer the trials of living in this evil world. There is one major advantage of having adopted children. They are already here. They are already living in our convoluted mess of a civilization. Do you notice how we responsibly screen and examine adopted and foster parents for suitability? We expect them to deliver the child a sustained, improved quality of life. We expect emotionally stable, well adjusted, materially able people to apply for the job of Parent. This seems responsible and pragmatic to us.

Children are not just going to take care of themselves. In effect, we want to protect the adopted child from possibly unfit parents. We are all in agreement. The holy people ask of us to pretend sex is the last thing on our minds and theirs. Consider this global insanity relating to matters of sex. Just look at the fascinating availability of venereal disease. See, the religious people have an excellent point. Is there something wrong with behavioral traits like responsibility, moderation, love, care, respect, concern, circumspection, kindness, and honesty? Do religious people have to apologize when they are right?

A fact is a fact. Sinful, irresponsible, self-indulgent, sexual behavior causes untold grief to children and adults alike. It can't be conducive to the health of the unborn to become born compromised with Acquired Immunodeficiency Syndrome, Gonorrhea, syphilis, Hepatitis, Human Papillomavirus (HPV). Is it more moral to allow the use of a condom?

It is clear. Sexual malpractice is counterproductive, to the security of adults and children alike. As a society seeks to regulate itself, it should remain beholden to solving problems already here. Contraception is nothing more than preventative medicine. The side effects of condom use seem minimal, when compared to a sick baby or adult. From a purely economic standpoint. A pack of condoms from the gas station saves multiple thousands in lifetime, medical costs. For a few disposable dollars in whatever currency, we can immediately save a child from an absent father. Why would the head of the home and society be missing in action on childcare and child support? That a male can leave his offspring solely in the hand of the weaker vessel defies logic. We would expect the dominant male to lead the parade on contraception. It would be expected. Males would use their socially approved status as a leader and ensure prophylactic use.

How is contraception use evil? We call our peculiar hypocrisy, a moral necessity, and it lays the matter to rest. Where is the love, the care, the concern, the overwhelming primal concern, for the innocent and vulnerable? We are busy to dignify a simple act of sexual intercourse, with marriage, relationships and pregnancy. This is a dangerously disproportionate investment, for a very transient attempt at pleasure. Contraception is a problem because it prevents women from being pregnant. Society compromises somewhat, its approved sexist power structure, with little innovations like birth control.

See Saudi Arabia. The year is 2016 C.E. Witness the car, as a means of social control. This is hardly a conspiracy theory. If you want to know where your girls are, please don't let them drive. There is always a social agenda. Laws, historically, are enacted to promote, protect, or suppress. There must be an agenda, because all life is agenda-driven. It is obvious from our history. The care and happiness of children is no cornerstone of our social agenda. In the bid to manage our women, we need the threat of pregnancy to always loom large. We are supposedly a rational life form, with a capacity for objectivity. It is a probable hope that our social agendas are honest & fair.

Human beings are usually fertile. We have the option to plan our children's life intelligently. We behave as if the gift of life amounts mainly to giving birth to male descendants. The denial of access to contraception and abortion is a propaganda devised to pretend at respect for and care for life. We know of the much-published regard some governments have for their military personnel. Just don't get wounded, and don't get captured, and whatever you do don't get stressed, and never lose the war. Usually, the government's devotion ends there. Children are routinely born to canceled care and non-existent welfare. To deceive the unborn, about their legitimate expectations for love, is exceptionally cruel. It is betrayal from conception.

The unborn need desperate access to the contraception being denied. Since females are the ones capable of being pregnant, any time we deny contraception, we deny it to a woman. Should we care? Who cares? They are only women. The unborn, even the female ones, still are entitled to our sympathy. We know adult women are terrible. We know of their capacity for (VMB) vicious, murderous bitching. Let us not insist they raise children against their wishes. Contraceptives including morning-after pills for women? Yes. The ayes have it.

God has not commanded to be fruitful and multiply, in any old style. God has not required of us, we fill and overfill the earth with hungry humanity. We know at least two world religions which expect the Almighty to intervene in earthly affairs and clean up the mess. Jesus is coming again. Why? It seems reasonable to conclude this present world system is compromised. Why do we insist others be born into the cesspool? Has Jesus Christ ever directed us to crowd our homes and cities, and to add daily and prodigiously to the ranks of the lonely, the abandoned, the enslaved, and the sexually exploited? Can we say Christ has moved us to swell with abandon our bellies, so those of the children can go empty? Has Christ commanded us to multiply exceedingly, so he can have more misery to fix on his return? We stamp the children, born, and then we abandon to hunger for the worst.

We want adults and teenagers to learn to be responsible parents on the baby's time. We want the big people to prove their maturity and commitment on the little people's time. Life is sacred. Pregnancy is sacred. We are sending raw recruits on a special ops mission. Hey, bunch of high-schoolers, here are some really good guns and night vision. Go take out Bin Laden. Don't worry, the ride is free. As long as society receives new citizens intact, we stop worshipping life. We should be ashamed to credit any such foolish plan to God. If this is God's plan, then God is a fool... like philandering Zeus. Has our God commanded us to pay the lowest wages possible, have the minimum safety standards, cut down the great forests of the earth, pollute the air and the waters, and crowd into slums and shanties in our quest to prosper?

Christ says, when a man comes to build a tower he should first consider the cost, to see if he will have sufficient funds to complete it. Lest when he has laid the foundation, he cannot complete his project, and passersby's mock his lack of planning and foresight. Jesus then exhorted his followers, "Therefore, you also count the cost." As you will notice the foundation is not the house. Conception is the foundation of a human being. The materials to build are there. Not by any means is the product the same as the very process itself. Do we see any respect for this cost-counting principle? The recommended absurdity is always procreation, never contraception. Child-rearing is a personal decision. It should remain just that. Personal.

The issue is not what is the optimal family size? The issue

is this. Civilized society should politely refrain from legislating children into birth. Our collective arrogance is overwhelming. Citizens of our global village blow babies to indiscriminate bits. These same kind hearts speak of morality, and decency, and law, and order. Worst still, we speak of right and wrong. The unborn are being bludgeoned into living. They are not being blessed into life. In what few wars has the civilian trauma, not exceeded the military casualties? Ok, the Pig War of 1859. We cannot aspire to make death an inconvenient necessity, only when we wish to wage our patriotic wars, or enforce public crackdowns.

Only our God knows what the future is. We are just making our best guess for our children, based on today's very incomplete data. And the data is always very much incomplete. Just ask history. As we know, all businesses need new customers. Religions need new adherents, just like the State, to pay taxes and to resist the encroachment of rivals. God presently has only one begotten son. And some major religious figures, as far as we know, have none. Somewhere from this zone of pediatric austerity, some still manage to oppose contraception. How can the rhythm method be any holier than condom use? We are deliberately and with intent attempting to prevent a pregnancy. Without doubt, I want us to continue with our rhythms and succeed.

All birth control is artificial. Artificial either in product or by design. All pregnancies are artificial, except for the miraculous types like the Virgin Mary. Women are not born with pregnancies loaded into them. How can contraception be a moral felony or misdemeanor? We conceive misery and call it a family. Is it sensible to burden ourselves with a marriage, a job, a career, a child, and then say it is the will of God? God's burden is light, so says his son Jesus Christ. Life is all about priorities. Can we pretend children don't daily curse their births? These child veterans go mostly unheeded and disregarded. It is not typical to shampoo the patient's dirty hair before we treat the gangrenous leg. Show a commitment of love to those already born, and earn permission to speak, about the imagined plight of not being born. It is usually illegal to incite others to criminal acts. Child abuse is a criminal act. By our standards, it is criminally insane to demand the delivery of children into our confusion and crisis.

This is a world at war. We pause only to reload. And to breed reinforcements. The embarrassment we are supposed to feel over sex is of ancient origins. In Genesis, we learn that God created and placed man nude in Eden. God encourages them to pursue the orgasm. God encouraged Adam and Eve to have sex and produce offspring. All the other animals were making out except for Adam. Humm, hum, hum, hum. It could not be the forbidden fruit. Our debilitating issues with nudity and sex are of our obsessive design. Why would a man and his wife feel uncomfortable being naked with each other? There was no pornography, no illegal drugs, no drunkenness, no taxes, and our first parents already were sexually dysfunctional. There was no one else in the room, and Adam and Eve were having body shaming issues. Adam and Eve aborted the quality of life their children would inherit. Having children never rectified that fundamental error.

After man disobeyed God, we see that Adam and Eve acquired another perspective on sex and nudity. We can't blame God for that. Because we can't come to grips with human sexuality, we absolutely cannot objectively deal with the downstream issues of reproduction. All these centuries later, we are still busy speaking about wardrobe malfunctions. We know one society's modest dress is a whore's costume in another. We have a tainted jury on the sex case. The Jury hates the fact it is well hung, but it is. Society can be uncompromising, unrelenting in its bid for conformity. No wonder Jesus came to set us free.

Reasonable people would suspect parenthood is a choice, not a social mandate. Pregnancy is a high-risk mission. Becoming someone's child is downright suicidal. It is astounding to the civilized mind, just how our bodies and our fertilities belong to the society itself. There is a context, where matters of reproduction become a matter needing regulation by the State.

The job of the State is to ensure, the contraceptives produced meet an appropriate standard of safe functionality. The job of the State is to ensure, doctors are qualified to meet the medical need of patients. Since the State is not itself a doctor, appropriately knowledgeable professionals will handle the empirical data. The State has the power to make any foolish or oppressive law it wishes. The historical data seems to beg for more, not less contraception.

The matter for us is not what the law is. The basis for our questions is what we know about children, and the society they get born into. Paralysis cannot claim our capacity to be rational, honest, and objective. The State must find it more reasonable to ban reproduction than to ban abortion. Contraception and abortion bans would be a legitimate social issue. It would be so, if human beings had a genetic obligation to reproduce at set intervals. From age fifteen, women would automatically produce a child every two years until age forty- one. Human beings really could have made it simple, by just having a regular breeding season. We would say that God, or nature, had so predetermined reproduction. It does not work this way.

Reproduction is a wee bit more involved. We put another person in harm's way. This is our unilateral decision. We are having a baby. This resonates as amoral and highhanded. We have, supposedly, in our deliberate judgment chosen to introduce a non- combatant, a juvenile, into our adult complications. We have to seek a willing, or unwilling fellowman to conceive. We have to seek conception. Interestingly, the fate of our offspring is out of our control. This seems very cavalier and extraordinarily proud, if not selfish, and downright evil. Who is playing God now?

Every conception is an artificial dictate. We manipulate ourselves into reproduction. We decide, or not decide, when new human terrors form. The unborn urge us to accept life is more than respiration. The unborn beg for the chance to visit us, when we are better able to receive them. The unborn will always be unborn. It is quite a bit of hubris to sentence people to life on this earth. There is no rush to invite new guests to our labor party. We insist humans have a choice to only procreate. This is no choice at all. It is a fraud of fact.

People will, or should always have rational, and prudent decisions to make about bearing children. Reproduction is not a self-perpetuating eventuality, or precondition of nature. Reproduction is a consequence impacting the unborn. We pretend the conception of a child is any more natural than the use of contraception. Both activities result from deliberate human conspiracy. A female's period is normal. Menstruation is natural for a woman. Pregnancy is artificial.

Unbothered by male incursions, a female would shed eggs until menopause. Simple. The overlords should dedicate to ensuring women have uninterrupted, comfortable menstruations. This seems to be the natural dictates of the female human body. Bleed, then stop. Provide subsidized iron tablets, hormone supplements, sanitary napkins, and medications which assure a regular menstrual cycle. The emphasis cannot be on pregnancy. Not one woman has yet been born, with the normal capacity to impregnate herself. Pregnancy is an artificial disruption of a very natural menstrual cycle. The implications of this artificial disruption extends past the mother. Childbirth is not as natural as we make it out to be.

We are not even going to delve into the numbers of females who have died during childbirth, or miscarried. Pregnancy has never been child's play. Pregnancy is an inherently unsafe and vulnerable time for women. Where are our law-makers, and religious leaders, when we need them? Ban pregnancy! It is an unnecessarily high risk and hazardous procedure. It seems irresponsible, considering the associated risks, to encourage females to bear children. Remember, the risk of death is totally in the female domain. To force or make childbirth inevitable is unconscionable.

Where exactly do males derive this moral authority to dictate terms of reproduction? Examine the unbiased, natural evidence. We pretend to be so practical and straightforward, even as we hijack fellow humanity with our laws and prejudices. Observe a woman, from the day of her birth to the day of her death. Unless her pet name is Mary, we may never see another baby divinely conceived. We choose to have children.

How immodest it is to see our kings, queens, rulers and law slink into our very private parts, to legislate their philosophies of living. How rude, how unnatural, how contrived, how creepy. It is improper to have your fellow humans legislate their way into your most sanctioned private moments. Reproduction. It is disgusting to think of this penile, vaginal voyeurism, as legally approved behavior. It is perverse, this legislative approval of Tom peeping. It is clear, just who the sexually twisted and deranged are? It is no surprise. Some of us, most obsessed with its legislation and regulation, perpetrate some of the worst sexual transgressions.

We are to be discussing the quality of life of a child, instead we find distraction in the sexual mores of the mother. Good, perhaps we should not force her to be a mommy now. The perspective is oppressive. Why else is it still necessary for Mary, the mother of Christ, to be a virgin? Poor deprived Joseph. Missionaries made and make endless forays into the uncivilized world to preach the Gospel, civilize the pagans, and to cover the heathen. This sexual embarrassment encourages some to view sex as evil, when consumed outside of wedlock, or without the inevitable conception of a child. We must not attempt to avert pregnancy. In other words, it is evil to enjoy sex as an end in itself. It is like eating only when you are hungry, and not one unnecessary calorie more. We are sick in the brain stems.

The pursuit of body-based righteousness is the ultimate vanity. Why should the mandatory conception of a child, or marriage occupy your mind, as you kiss, suck, stroke, thrust, touch, squeeze, lick, laugh, squirm, gyrate, moan, grunt, smile, giggle, encourage, suggest, and caress? Why must sexual intercourse become a communally regulated activity? The world is an oppressive place. So ordinarily oppressive.

This world basks in its power to control the minds and

actions of its citizens. We should be cautious about conceiving a child to inherit slavery. We would be wise about being addicted to sexual pleasure and interaction. Why? The major problem with sex is there are other people involved. Sex will always only be as good as the people involved in the act. The runaway obsession with sex is not healthier than the stifled self-smothering of the hypocritical and misguided. As with all things physical, sex is much ado about nothing. We come, it goes. That our bodies are the temple of God should put it all in perspective.

We are punishing unborn humans, because we have problems with our sexuality. Our lusts, they torment us. We usurp the personal space. We are oppressive. It takes a rapist to crawl into a woman's vagina and compel her to accept his will. We have entire state legislatures, and religious bodies forcing their way up to the cervix. This must hurt. Talk of no Vaseline. Talk of being sexually abused and traumatized. There is a patriotic front dedicated to denying the unborn the very prospect of a stable future. Everybody who becomes pregnant is not ready to be a parent.

We wrap all our adult issues into a cause exclusive to the unborn. We have women's rights, religious dogma, and ambitions, we have issues of morality; we have our political ambitions, and racial, and social stereotypes to account for. We are our contamination of the process. Contraception is about saving unborn lives. Abortion? What is abortion? Have we never heard of contraception? Yes, we have a choice.

We sometimes use the story of the biblical Onan, to show contraception is wrong and sinful. The Genesis story is straightforward. Onan had the duty of levirate to accomplish. He knew the heir would not be his. When he had sex with his deceased brothers' wife, he successfully decided on the highly unreliable withdrawal method and deprived his dead brother of an heir. Talk of pathological covetousness. It strains even the mind of a fool, to conclude God's displeasure was with contraception. Onan's selfishness upset God. Typically, we enjoy the spoils and forget our duties. Intent is everything with God. Intent. Motive. Attitude. Onan displeased God. Onan had his fun, and still felt it necessary to defraud Tamar, of the heir he had married Tamar to produce, in her dead husband's name.

It displeased God that Jacob treated Rachel's sister Leah as second class wife. How sensitive God is. The moral of the story. God regards not only the act but also more critically the motive prompting the act. This explains, "If you give your body to be burnt, and you have not love it profits you nothing." We should know by now that killing is neither here nor there. Why do we kill when we kill? Why do we make financial donations? Why do we get married? Why did we have children? Why did we retire from our job? Why? Why did we offer this or that person our help? Why did we conceive a child, why, why, why? The act of withdrawal is not the issue. If coitus interruptus is sinful, then so is the rhythm method and abstinence. The mindset, which motivated the act upset God. Some have been partial in recent times to natural contraception, meaning the rhythm method. Do we see withdrawal to be anything but natural? We have often spoken of hypocrisy. This procreation prerequisite is hypocrisy. It is used to disguise our distaste for, and our discomfort with pure, raw, or steamed sexual passion.

How does the prevention of conception, by keeping male sperm from the female egg, become an evil deed? As we have pointed out before, it upsets somebody couples enjoy sex for the fun of it. It is sexually immoral for persons outside the marital bed, to make group sex out of reproduction. This communal regulation of sexual activity is most disconcerting. The whole idea seems perverted and extraordinarily intrusive. Just when you thought you had a little private time to relax, the long arm of the law is fondling its perversions, and on your time. This malignancy is a blight on our societies. It is burdensome to the point of neurosis. Some behaviors are not polite.

We are still debating the morality of condom use, even for the lawfully wedded. The biological reality of Sexually Transmissible Disease does, however, make condom use almost synonymous with non-monogamous sexual activity. You can see how backward the whole notion of contraception is. We do not even have fertilization, and we are already condemning persons for destroying potential human life. Alternatively, do we wish to promote immoral pregnancies, because of unprotected intercourse? If the point of marriage is to raise children, then we must protect this institution. Ensure no children are conceived out of wedlock. Stoning comes immediately to mind.

The Western world needs to stop calling other cultures barbaric. As we can see, the Taliban and ISIS agree with our sexual prejudices. They are just more efficient at maintaining order. The sexually active must regard contraception seriously, if we desire to save the unborn any of the pain of abortion. Abortion is so very much a mostly preventable disease.

Contraception is essential to save the life of the unborn. Contraception helps ensure the children we have, are the ones we always wanted. Contraception does not make decisions. It cannot inherently be good or evil. End if you wish the debate. Satanists use the Holy Bible in rituals. Satan quotes it all the time. Are we then to regard the Bible as evil? Every day of the week, we misquote and misuse the Holy Word. It should remain legitimate, and the teachers, scholars, priests, preachers, writers, and pastors, I would suppose, remain evil and illegitimate.

Contraception helps fulfill that need for intelligently conceived offspring. Just one little sperm spill can create large ripples of responsibility and misery. We should hasten to the sterilization table. The sterilization table is a definite help in avoiding the abortion table. We cannot be casual about destroying unborn life. The abortion drama is very avoidable. Abortion is organically opposed to the business of raising children.

It is our sacred duty to evade the need for abortions. It is our most basic duty to produce our children with professional dedication. Our children will appreciate the concern. We misguide ourselves to claim the abortion event as constitutional freedom. Abortion is about children's rights to willing parents, not women's rights to reproductive choice. Very separate issues intertwined by the inconvenience of physical proximity.

Let life not end with abortion. Let life begin with contraception.

CONTRACEPTION CRUSADES & HOLY WARS

The Authorities wish to protect the health of women. We agree. Let's be proactive and reform our social breeding program. Required are major reforms to more effectively protect the health of women and the unborn. We must conduct mandatory testing for sexually transmitted diseases before we permit sexual intercourse. This, qualified health officials will handle in approved facilities. Then there should be a four day waiting period to confirm the desire for coitus. A registered phycologist should be on hand, in case persons require post-coital counseling. Law enforcement resources should be within fifteen minutes response time. This covers eventualities, such as abuse arising after consent.

We all accept that the religious laws against adultery exist because it occurs. Sexual immorality within wedlock is particularly dangerous. The use of protective devices, such as condoms, may be unlikely because of the fidelity expected. Religious persons, especially, should understand the need for regular testing, before intimate act occurs. Christians know, the scripture says, the heart of man is deceitful and desperately wicked. "Thou shalt not commit adultery" is not there for good looks.

Our faith in the word of God should lead us to appreciate the real possibilities. We could infect our spouse and our babies with a sexually transmitted disease. The government should manage our sexual contacts, with the same interest they manage our pregnancies and our access to contraception. Couples duly monitored for compliance would enjoy less frequent screenings. The health of the mother and child, as always, remains central to our concerns. The State should continue to revel in its management of our private family affairs, not to mention improved financial support. The basic financial package, for childcare, should border at least near lower middle class.

It is September 12th, 1994. It is the 12th because yesterday was September the 11th. The world population conference is going on in Cairo, Egypt. Some clerics objected to the conference and deemed holding it on Islamic soil illegal. They purported that it violated Islamic principle. The consensus view of these clerics was that abortion was wrong. This is a reasonable legal and moral issue, needing careful consideration. The Prophet Mohammed ruled that a man might have no more than four wives. The Prophet was himself allowed a more privileged number. As we see special circumstances can yield exceptions to the general rule. Mohammed specified a man had to provide his four wives financial support and equal marital access. A man could not appropriate a wife in any irresponsible way. He did not say the man had to be wealthy. A man had to understand his capability, in the present tense. It is necessary, we see, for an Islamic man to practice responsible wife control. It would evade reason for child (birth) control, to be a concept foreign to Islamic principle.

Everywhere, physical matters need some management. Even while we debate the spiritual implications of birth management, misery promises to fill universal space. Poverty and hunger are pandemic. Why insist a child be born, so we can show him or her, the wonders of scavenging for food and rags in the city dumps? There are entire multitudes, of children, born to be wards more like prisoners of the State. There are multitudes more born to be untouchables. Untouchable. That is what we call a gift of life. I use obvious examples to make it simple. Every child who had hell's angels for parents, not the bikers, know the tension they call childhood and adolescence. Gulags come in a variety of zip codes, and climates.

If we have a steady job at the company, why rush to conception mode. A job is a job. It belongs to the person hiring. Where is the source of our security? We do our best and some cross fingers, and some pray. Children hate to inherit debt and hunger. Children prefer when their parents are kings, queens and princesses and princes. This however ends badly quite a few times. Ask British King Charles I, French Queen, Marie Antoinette, or the more recently deceased Russian Czar Nicholas II. Whatever the uncertainties, we know this. Children need care.

I must admit financial independence is a trick requirement. We can guarantee nothing, not our safety, not our spouse's availability, not our wealth, or the lack of it. At the very least, we can use our current circumstances as a guide in our reproductive ambitions. The stock market preaches this message daily. Humility should therefore assure us into quietness. We are not the demigods we imagine we are. We are easily distressed, and our plans set to naught. We should exercise great caution with the decisions we make about the lives of others. We owe the unborn this little courtesy. We should not allow social pressure to bully our children into reluctant birth.

We say and know the world is not perfect. Aha. Considering the precarious and doubtful nature of life, we would happily invest the very best of our available uncertain moments into our children. Family life demands inordinate amounts of time. Family life, if not encouraged to flourish, dies miserably. We know that. If we do not own our lives, there is very little of nothing left to share with our offspring. Do we live in daily regard of layoffs, of the manager's mood, fear of the police, of deadlines, and wage freezes? Do we owe the bank, the store, and our parents-in-law? Kids hate that. Children do not take kindly to handling economic stress. This is an exclusively adult option. When we have a child, we are taking a chance with someone else's life. Most people have lost enough gambling not to count themselves lucky.

It is clear. We have lost the population lottery. Multitudes of bankrupt lives. Yet we compel one and all to play yet another round of baby roulette. We do not qualify to insist, when other people have children. We are being big, bad, burly bullies. Exposing and quantifying all the misery children suffer, does not annul the pain and deprivation. It only shows we have talented researchers. The abandoned child is abandoned. The child slave is a child slave. The child prostitute is a child prostitute. The burnt child is burnt. The abused child is abused. The file on that child is a file. What we review on the video has already tragically occurred.

Moral people sometimes advocate marriage as a cure for the ills of abortion. This is fine. All we need to understand is the unborn will always need contraception and abortion services. Married couples also have these moral decisions to make regarding the wellbeing of their offspring. I know we love marriage and having a special friend. Some folks even like to think it quaint that polygamy is a legal option. I sort of oppose polygamy because I struggle to understand the use of monogamy.

Marriage is an adult relationship and construct. Marriage does not necessarily qualify us to be parents. A baby is someone else's life in our hands. We always have baby decisions to make, heedless of our marital status. The problem with polygamy or polyandry is not the number of wives or husbands. The problem with polygamy is marriage inequality. In this post-slavery era, it is no less demeaning to be the sole inferior wife as opposed to being one of many. When people respect each other, it matters not how we label the cohabitation, except for the legal convenience. Marriage is an excellent tool for navigating our societies. What happens to the children when we think the spouse is no longer good enough for us? What is the unborn to say?

Love is love. It is, or it is not. Jesus came to set us free. He said according to the record. Love one another. Contrary to the Western outlook. Arranged marriages provide women with at least one disclaimer. The society is responsible for their social circumstance. In the West, we are so free. How does a progressive, modern female squander her freedom to become the number two in class? How does an individual accept the statutory and social subjection required by the marriage covenant? Marriage, as an institution of convention, has proven itself a squalid, outdated, unkind human tradition. Lastly, how can an adult be so naïve as to believe the words, "I love you?" Marriage traditionally countenances, promotes and demands inequality, slavery, and serfdom. Lastly, you need permission for divorce usually.

This is not exactly the best pasture for our children. I won't dare suggest marriage as automatically good family business. Notwithstanding my dislike. The intent of marriage is good, and much superior to children strewn around the fertile crescent. Childbirth essentially and unambiguously requires a willing mother. Everybody deposits genetic material for conception. Only one person incubates life and possibly dies in childbirth.

Life is a pure science. If we don't want to hurt the babies, we can choose not to have them. This is abstinence & contraception. If the babies will get hurt, we reduce their suffering as much as possible. This is abortion. If we don't mind the gamble, we bring the pregnancy to term. This is childbirth. We all inherit ourselves. The seminal issue is, where is the child's caretaker? We cannot serve two masters. We cannot serve the traditions and the reality. As a matter of self-preservation, I believe in freedom. As an unborn child, I choose willing, ready parents.

Children are looking for stability and continuity. They don't care how we define the sexual arrangement. Children seem to like their committed parents to be together, in harmony. Marriage itself does not qualify us to be parents. Marriage is a token of our commitment to love one another as ourselves. You need not marry to love. Marriage itself is not love. Imagine. You might not want to have another baby with your very husband or wife. The same one you would divorce or dispose of in a heartbeat, if only you could. Well, the unborn baby is taking notes and filing an abortion application.

Man riddles with bullet points a history of violence, betrayal, and pain, oppression, inequality, brutality, and the occasional calm. No civilized, individual, or society should be so pompous, as to compel reproduction. We speak of abortion and murder. Giving birth may well be genocide. Why are we as adults, so young? Why all the vain pretensions? Regard the toxic human reality we dwell in? We seek to evade our responsibility to human life, by the childbirth mandate. Who do we think we are? How proud, how cowardly, how arrogant, how hypocritical.

Some of us regard any discussion concerning a decline in the African birth rate, to be racist. It is thought, birth control is a white ploy, to depopulate Africa again, and make it vulnerable to recolonization. Admittedly, black Africans must carefully examine all nice suggestions, originating from Caucasia. This time, just this time, we might want the whites to succeed, with their little ploy. We have surrendered to worst ideas than contraceptive use. Like Ph.D.'s in Scooby Doo and Tom and Jerry.

We must be careful to agree that a black child is as important as any other. Black lives matter. There is no need to make abortion an issue of race. Children need parents, committed to being parents. There is no race card to play with abortion. Not unless white people are forcibly destroying the pregnancies black people wish to keep. Then this would be no game. Abortion means we do not want a baby. No baby should have to be born to parents until the parents at least think it is a magnificent idea. This is the black and white truth.

Abortion is about children, not marital status, approved social sex prejudice, or fantasies of faith, or near Utopia. Every abortion has its own story and circumstance. It is personal. Our children require a future vastly superior to the one we offer. A great sin it is, to play religious politics with the fate of the children. To this day, our commitment to our children remains basic. From day one, we notify our newborn children, "I brought you into this world. I have done my bit. Now you're on your own. You owe me." Couples have the choice to create or, not create a larger family. Most like to extend the family. First tire our ear, before you cease to let us hear; parenting is a tiresome business. Children do not appreciate it when we cut corners in designing their future. Not that they will appreciate the efforts. The most severely regulated industry should be the baby industry. What the pious powers seem to require is the unhindered birth of yet another unwanted, or situationally compromised child.

We expect only qualified architects to build our homes and bridges. Any two old fools can produce a baby. We speak so confidently about the sanctity of life. The reverence we claim for human life disappears when we become buried in mountains of discounted humanity.

Explosives better have expert manufacture, or we face much uncertainty as to the future or immediate stability of the product. No such regard for competence occupies us when we create another life. When things blow up, well, we did the best we knew how to. Despite the mini and mass detonations of lives improperly formulated in childhood and adolescence, every day, more family amateurs have children. Since the situation grows on caressed, we can conclude we are quite pleased with our activities. We have created oceans of baby tears, entire atmospheres full of loneliness, cloud loads of despondency, and a variation of everything depressing and painful.

Maternity wards continue to be among the most visited areas on earth. Males remain exuberant about the ability to squirt fertile sperm. The statisticians attempt to document and quantify the folly, however, grief expands at, and surpasses the speed of light. Incredibly, we will die for our children, we will die because of them, but we refuse to live for them.

The tears of our children alert us. We must regulate more stridently the expression of our various fertilities. The loneliness reflects from our children's eyes in bright, uncluttered images. If time is not an abundant resource, our children will wait to be born until it is. Please, don't force the child to inherit for all time a miserable human for his parent. We have failed very well as parents. We don't hate our children. We are just tired of the little ignorant brats. Yes, we are tired.

Let's consider more of our abortion resistant landscape. Raising children is not prestigious, glamorous, or fulfilling enough to be a career. Are we the same people, busy ensuring others become parents? What then is so valuable about these precious microscopic babies three days after conception? It is a precious human life. The irony of it all. Children are not farms, they need parents, not just assigned help. Yes, we are tired. Let us be clear. Does being a stay-at-home parent create an identity crisis for us? Are we sure we're old enough? Not just to have children, but to be parents? Parents are gods.

It is hardly as exacting a process to run for president or prime minister. Your marriage may be in disarray, your family life in shambles, and you can still be an efficient and well-loved president. Parenthood does not allow for such liberties or indulgences. The children are in our faces, from delivery. Children ultimately diet on parental vibes. The historical unhappiness, which pervades the marriage covenant, assures us. We are not as ready for childbearing as we think. If we set even modest standards for parenting, we would easily see.

We would see how tragic it is to legislate a new life into this world. Where is our empathy? Where is our pragmatism? Where are our street smarts and our doctorate degrees? Where is our sense of reality, and where is our wisdom? We should not punish immorality, by whipping it into submission, with a live, bawling, milk craving baby. We can help by not being immoral ourselves.

Is marriage a license to procreate pain? Human marriage is the expensive purchase of the hope of exclusive sexual activity, with the man usually on top. It is a pain-creating fallacy that being married is of itself, enough to warrant childbearing. How does that which is riddled, and potholed with anxiety, hatred, dislike, and hurt, fail to offer its children the same as a comforter? There are many ways to provide social support for children, other than the nuclear family. The undying question is this. Should the society compel someone to become a career caregiver, when they would rather not be such?

How does society compel you to be a parent? There is an unborn child involved in this compelling, lifelong saga. There are consequences of giving birth. Why does such a generous society, not compel you to be wealthy, at its own expense? How can children reap, from their parents, a joy which was never sown? It may please the religious community to see any decline in the divorce rate. This hardly indicates a rise in the joy rate within the marriage community. A weighty act conception is. We are creating a new human life because we wish it. Where are my parents? The conceived want to know. We know God probably did not command you to have the child, any more than he commanded you, to marry Mr. Otywack. Did God also command us to be a farmer, or a banker, or a bank robber, or a nurse, or a politician? The command is to love one another as self. Love also inexplicably knows no law. Love is so real, a list of do and don'ts cannot contain it. As Paul says, if the Law could have worked and supplied righteousness, it would have.

Let us go back to the universally exported story of Adam and Eve. The first dysfunctional parents in history. As we recall, all was fine in the Garden of Eden. An abundance of the environmentally, pristine, exotic pets, and a surplus of non-genetically modified foods. In particular, there was the Tree of Life. Not a tree of life, the Tree of Pro-life. Adam and Eve were already alive, why would they need any more life? We know the story. Adam and Eve ended up being very much dead, while alive. Our children need more than birth. The unborn need adults willing to feed them life.

Mercy forbids, we bear a child to see if she will help keep our marriage together. This is a very bizarre arrangement. Parents must smooth out the cloths of their marital bed, before conceiving a little bundle of joy to share it. We insist on bringing the unborn into our world. We are certain our wife is now bitching incarnate, or the husband transformed into a worthless liability. All the child wants to know for now is, "Who will take care of me?"

Adults flee the terror of other adults. Adults migrate, they hike deserts and snow-clad peaks, and they despair even to suicide. Adults die at the hands of their loving, lawfully wedded spouses. Adults lose their minds, from the intricate tortures lavished on them, by loving, lawfully wedded spouses. Adults despair and die. Adults despair and shrivel in marriage's loving embrace. Somehow we expect children to shrug off the abuse, the darkness, the contentions, the suffocation, and blossom into God's little angels. Miracle indeed.

The concept of abortion to this day remains a pariah notion. The indiscriminate, avoidable slaughter of millions of the unborn assaults our humanity. It should. The fact is. Some unborn children have an urgent need for abortion. We all have our urgent medical needs. We the children want more abortion access, even as we want fewer abortions. We the unborn need simpler access to medical abortions. Most of all, we need our contraceptives.

As we might suspect. Abortion is not about marital status. Children want willing, loving parents. No child, to our knowledge, has yet made this explicit request from the womb. We just assume on their behalf that this is their true desire. Contraception should hold good, righteous symbolism for us. Contraception shines, a healthy sun, on the pallor of abortion's deaths. For contraception to work, we have to stop regarding pregnancy as a reasonable byproduct of sexual intercourse.

It is foolish to create a child to share our marital insecurities. We persist in being pregnant. To rip an unborn child from the womb is barbaric. To rip an unborn child (from the blissful separateness of his mother's egg and father's sperm), to inherit sterility is humane, understandable, and reasonable. Please remember, all the terrible people we so freely gossip about are usually someone's parents. The backstabbing colleague on the job, the lying, tale-bearing associate at the office, the proverbial bitch, and these other terrible folks we just can't stand have children too. Are we not happy they use contraception sometimes?

We say human life, like it describes some magical state of well-being and contentment. Abortion remains relevant, mainly because we don't take good care of each other. The problem with abortion is, it usually solves a very unnecessary problem.

The jury is still out, accessing the failed and cancerous health of our notion of family. That jury is dishonest, lost, or foolish. If the jury is out, the evidence is in. The evidence is at home. The evidence is in jail. The evidence is in the cemeteries. The evidence is in family court. The evidence is in no care at all. The evidence is in and under our city streets, and the evidence is on the psychologist couch. The evidence is on the battlefield. The evidence unfortunately is in our very beds. The evidence is plentiful. The evidence is in government. It is in our separate minds and our individual lives. The evidence is so available. It is no burden at all to prove. We have burdened our children with every malignancy.

Abortion and childbirth occupy the same pregnant space. Our job as a society is indeed to preserve the uterine space, as a place to nurture, not kill babies. Attitudes matter. When consenting women find themselves with an unwanted pregnancy, the question is, "How did I fuck up?" Invoking a fundamental female right to an abortion is patently delirious; deliciously amoral, murderous, and egotistical. We know it is wrong when over-righteous zeal, converts a simple first-trimester abortion, into a late-term abortion, or no abortion at all. All the legislative roadblocks to early, swift, and prompt abortion are part and parcel of the murderous equation. There is a time for everything, even a time not to be born. Our purported humanity should spur us to spare the unborn babies the gift of unhappiness. Life can begin at contraception when you think of it.

Abortion is like dealing with a blaze. The fire department deals with the main issue at hand. Fire. They deal with extinguishing the blaze. It does not matter, at this exact point, whether the blaze was arson or accidental. Of course they would like to know. Let parents choose life, we don't force it on the child.

If unmarried sex is immoral or illegal, it should be easy for society to understand the need for abortion. Do we want a perfectly proper baby conceived from an act we despise? Is abortion more evil than being called bastard and illegitimate for all your life? Certainly though, abortion makes you more dead. Our societies are morally unfit to prevent legal access to abortion.

The unborn deserve either the prospects for a full life, or a premature death. For once, let us not show any balls, and let us show a little resolve. If we would show our balls less in the first place, then we would have fewer abortions to attend to. Let us resolve to stamp out in our lives, irresponsible human procreation. A few vasectomies may be helpful.

We know, apart from miscarriages, abortion is a contrived event. Like sexual intercourse. How would anyone stigmatize access to contraception? How would we, as decent people, claim abortion as a human right? Abstinence is not contraception any more than hunger is dieting. The technology is available, let it be available without judgment, and the social censure. Those who abstain do not need contraception. Those who indulge usually do. We should not deny the unborn access to both contraception and abortion. It seems a patently misguided policy.

We believe human beings have the authority to propagate human life, because it's so correct, easy, and so natural. Weeds spring perennially from the earth that sustains our agriculture. Weeds, like children, are so easy to grow, so natural. A little fertile soil and a little water. The conditions are simple but exact. It is a basic matter. For child propagation, can we give an eternal warranty on the joy, love, and peace? This would be so correct.

It seems unnecessary to convince men and women. Childbearing is a hefty and unpredictable responsibility. It seems so obvious. If we don't plan on being the absolute best parents we can be, don't we yet see why abortion works? Let us be kind to the babies.

If you will notice, all silly traditions deprive someone of joy. The tradition of the inferior woman deprives a woman of the benefits of her individuality, from the very instant of conception. Good girls can't even go to heaven, without their husband signing a consent form. The tradition God doesn't exist leaves us groping for answers, and solutions to questions already answered. The tradition of the superior white has given birth to that cancerous matrix of an enduring, active, lingering oppression on every continent. Embedded clusters of legacied, whitewashed hatred. The tradition, tradition is itself sacred and inviolate, is perhaps the most absurd of the traditions.

Babies are born to teenage children in the very sewers, which transport urbane shit. The children of the world dwell in emotional sewers. Where more appropriate for our children to dwell than in the sewers? We have a long tradition of treating them like shit.

Our humanity is not exactly shy, about generously sharing pain and hurt. Are we naturally duty-bound to create children to share our miseries? We know our husbands abuse us. We know adult women are oppressed. We continue to bear life upon life, into a situation we deem intolerable for adults. Our quaint cultural dainties result in girls being deprived of a clitoris. Well, children belong to their parents, alive or dead. Born or unborn. Our treasured cultural gems manifest themselves in the sewn up vaginas of little girls, all in the name of sexual purity. I think clitoris deprivation is, to say it appropriately, only the tip of the issue. Vain philosophy does more than blow hot air. The toxins of our beliefs manifest themselves tragically.

Women are to this day born, without an absolute claim to the very body they move around in. We take a dim view of this oppression. To our claim of abortion, as a fundamental female right, the unborn also take a dim view of this. Our unborn girls wonder aloud, "What exactly is their f@#k%$g problem with contraception?" To put it mildly, let the born be joyful, or let the unborn remain unborn.

SURVIVING THE FITTEST. THE NEXT TARGET

"The next target of those who support abortion is the elderly, the dependent, and others classified, as lacking the capacity for meaningful life." This is a valid concern. We know ideology directs our paths. Women don't sometimes get paid less, for the same work, because of clerical error. Philosophy directs our paths. Our perennial wars and annual civil conflicts confirm human beings kill, and cause death, with great regularity... even when we are at peace. Our appetite for each other dead is not a symptom of abortion poisoning. I was a little taken aback. Consider the human history of open criminal warfare. How is abortion the catalyst for and culprit in our heartlessness. We are born and sometimes we die of old age. Some of us also spend our last days senile, immensely handicapped, and utterly dependent. It is official. The authorities do not permit us to walk around, deciding when others should die. As reality would have it, people sometimes need help with living and with dying. We are hopeful those who must act on our behalf, would do so with love, or professionally at least.

We have concluded, rather self-righteously, and vainly I must add, that living is always in our interest. Once we have lost that discretion to manage our lives, our life goes from challenging to pathetic. It is always murder to dispose of a life, because we hate its owner. The elderly and others needing extra care and attention, remind me rather easily of newborn babes. One major difference is people usually see their children as desirable investments. Some need an heir, some need people to care for them in old age, some just like the attention of having children among other reasons. Some want a family.

As with abortion, we are quick to consume our attention with those who seek to evade caretaking responsibility. This time, we focus on young adults who abandon their aged parents, to everybody, anybody and sometimes to nobody at all. Again, the issue is not primarily the responsibility dodger. If your child does not want to take care of you. Well, we are speechless. Unlike unborn children, adults know about the perils of becoming sick, old, or disabled. It seems reasonable, we would all have our suicide option as a normal part of our life plan. The concern always lies with the quality of life a human being can endure or enjoy. Sometimes we need to employ the services of death. Civilized people don't murder people, we just cause each other to die. It is not unheard of that doctors have to make judgment calls about who will receive priority for life-saving attention.

The purpose of abortion is not to rid the earth of babies. It is useful to appreciate that. All dependant people need caretakers. Women have abortions because they don't want to be mothers. They may very well have jobs as caretakers, nannies even. If you don't want to care for a parent or dependant child, you abandon them. That's an option. If you wish to hasten your parents' death for material gain, this is another option. An elderly person differs from an unborn child. One has forged a life, and the other, lacking the essential knowledge of a life to be, is being incubated inside someone else. It is useful to understand just how ignorant a first-trimester baby is. We do not perform abortions as some vendetta against life. We perform abortions mainly because someone does not want to be a mom. Children naturally want to be born to parents who desire their birth.

Forever, man has been distraught by the uselessness of his achievements, and the anti-climactic suspension of his ration of time. Dreams of immortality and life's sanctity are our emotional balm. Our very selfish world pretends it holds life as sacred. Respect for the sanctity of life gets paid, as long as those in need of death die, without external help. There will always be people needing others to make life and death decisions on their behalf. This is the nature of life. Caretakers mostly do exactly what the word suggests. Care. They care for those who are incapable of caring for themselves.

Since the expectation is abortion will lead to the abuse of the dependent others, we must wonder. What happens to a dependent child who was born unwanted?

When alive we have the breath of life, but human life is infinitely superior to the mere breath of life. Human life is a personal manipulation of the breath of life. It is no toast to life to chain it to impotence. A mouse shares the air we breathe, but the agenda is mousey and routine: eat, procreate and die. The mouse, we believe, attaches no great significance to any of these activities. Man can attach whatever significance he desires to each and any activity. Man may emphasize, or neglect, any state, stage, or activity in her life. Man thinks, albeit badly. When we reduce life to the ability to respire, we desecrate the concept of life. The aging of our parents should encourage us to redeem the time. The clock stops. For a child to be born for abuse and deprivation is criminally insane. Life is worth the while, for a child, because it was family time well spent. If it were not for adulthood, many a child would be hopelessly and perpetually lost in that vortex of emotional rape and physical restraint.

People typically fear death, and those willing to kill. Death is naturally available and inevitable. When you destroy your attacker, you have not created an unnatural monster situation called death. You may just have destroyed an unnatural monster called murder. We must select carefully our motives when creating the death condition. The question why is a hallmark of true civilization. We want to know why what happened, not just what happened. What happens may be the grisly death of the defenseless unborn. Why did the death of the unborn occur? Why did we give birth, for example?

It always is the why. Why determines the morality or amorality of an action or situation. The Eternal God could have spared Jesus the reported drama on the cross. He did not. Why not? Suicide remains stigmatized, if not illegal. It is erroneous to make a blanket statement about taking one's life. Again motive. Jesus says: "Greater love has no man than he who would give up his life for his friend." Jesus knows what he is talking about. He gave up his life, to save those who were not his friends. Jesus knew that he would die; he waited for his murder. He aided and abetted his death, even asking that his disciples not suffer arrest. Jesus's death sounds nearly like a suicide by cop. Suicide by Roman legionnaire. Jesus with premeditation arranged for others to kill him. He, according to unknown sources, reportedly said in his defense, "They had a choice. I never forced them to murder me. I knew my murder was for the good of all mankind."

If fear or despondency motivates suicide, it is illegitimate. God says that. God wants us to fear him and nothing else. What motivates our suicide is however none of the State's business. Except if we owe the State information or taxes. What motivates your act of abortion is similarly not the business of the State. But you can share. Data helps shape policy. We must be careful to appreciate we have no authority, to conceive misery for others, including the unborn. If we choose to commit suicide, it is no great deal. Casually analyzed, we would have merely deprived ourselves of life. This leads us to the people who will drive you to suicide, so they can have the inheritance. It is hysterically contradictory that Western society, which is by virtue, agnostic, atheistic, and faithless, would make suicide a social offense. It is the spiritual spark, the invisible essences which gives us pause about death, and about giving life.

If the purpose of man's existence is to eat, drink, and be

merry, then there is absolutely no reason on earth to disapprove of suicide. The individual does not like our company, and so he or she skipped dinner and left early. It's as simple as checking out prematurely, because you hated your accommodation at the hotel. Only when we ingest suicide on a spiritual level, does it need self-regulation. It is an arrogant usurpation of the virtue of self-determination, for anyone to refuse you access to your death. Thou shalt not kill is a commandment of murder. We think we respect and honor life because we have killed no one. It is of no interest to us how our actions ruin the lives and livelihoods of others. How many people involved in destroying families think of themselves as murderers? Abortion is an easy target because people stop breathing.

The State can draft us into its army and send us to kill others on the battlefield. We also get to kill daughters and sons as collateral damage. The State encourages you to hate the enemy. The State promises to absolve you of all criminal liability for the deaths. We realistically ignore the motives of the individual soldiers causing the carnage, and we focus on the national good. We must protect ourselves, we say, even if it means the inadvertent destruction of children born and unborn. When you bomb a city, the death of civilians is a necessary auxiliary event, we agree. We allow necessary distress for the national agenda. We frustrate the doctrine of necessity on the personal level. Individual freedom, in matters of death, is too much independence for mere citizens. What if someday the State has free people to deal with? Well, this is a pragmatic concern.

Back to abortion. Why don't we walk into the maternity ward and snap the necks of the children born to abusive parents? I also consider the deformed, and the mentally retarded, who have long been born and are fixtures in our society. Why don't we walk up to them and kill them out of their misery? I feel these people have every right to continue to suffer the traumas of life if they so desire. I think. Why should I deny the unborn the chance to suffer through life, and take their chances with life? I was worrying along the line of an entirely fallacious premise. This is not and never should be my decision. It is not our job to cull human life. Sometimes, though, the death quandary will be in our jurisdiction. The decision we must make.

Unborn people, to put it indelicately, exist mostly in our imagination. All this stuff about aborted children not having the pleasure of seeing a sunset, or of falling in love, or of joining the KKK is whimsical nonsense. We can just as easily replace these dreams with any of the many horrors we are so well acquainted with. We seem truly unaware that babies do not care and nurture themselves. It is lunacy to talk, about unborn life, like it is some commodity which pops out independent and equipped. After nine months in the womb and baby is ready. Children need parents. Children don't gain parents because there is a law saying they ought to have two.

In the global context, though, we can always agree. Personal decisions relating to death will always have to be made. The children, who are already born, crave an improved living. A two-year-old baby is not unborn, and it is foolish to expect her abortion. Please understand. Women do not get pregnant so they can have a six hundred dollar abortion. Think of how much nail polish the sluts can buy with that dough. Typically, women who don't want to be mothers have abortions. The issue is about becoming a parent. You don't cure a lack of parenting desire by having a baby. Our commitment is to prevent the conception of family apathy. This is the virtue of abortion. It eliminates in the present the complications of the future. Now there is a time for every purpose under heaven.

The fact many children already live swaddled in emotional deprivation is proof. We have failed in our commitment and duty. The existence of shantytowns does not validate their proliferation. "Shall we continue in sin that grace may abound?" Individuals who are already born are born. Does not their plight sway us to the need to prevent the creation of such misery in the first place? When your baby is born, you are duty-bound to find her joy, or she should have found an early death. When your baby is born, he is no longer unborn. We do not abort after birth.

As a fact, the authorities restrict most legal abortions to under twenty- four weeks. A most reasonable balance between the interests of the non-cooperative parent and our future adult.

Partial-birth abortion is the ultimate misnomer. Partial-birth abortion may be murder, euthanasia, or whatever, but it is not the abortion of a birth. What happens to a baby after she is born? This is another decision to make. The child after birth is squarely now in the public domain. The society now has a greater legitimate right to police every breath taken. There is a moral, present, and prudent jurisdiction to protect. What level of interference is expedient, tolerable, reasonable is another social debate. I vote against the very concept of unrestricted abortion. Late-term abortion reinforces the misconception that women own a right to kill the unborn. Abortion is an unsatisfactorily negotiated compromise.

Death is a lifelong reality. Death decisions don't confine themselves to the pregnancy state. Whenever someone is entrusted with the care of our decisions, we must choose joy. Consider you have a newborn baby, whom you dislike. You are unwilling, or unable, to produce joy in that child's life. Consider you abdicate your responsibilities as a parent. To whom? He is your child. Consider that no one else is willing or able to accept the charge for the child. Still, she is your child. The child needs love and friendship, not just breakfast, and a bed in a Socialist funded orphanage. That child long deserved the love of life, or the peace of death. It was our decision. Who had to make that life or death decision? You.

If we give birth to a responsibility, should we not accept it? We conceive a child we know needs love. We know our reserves of that essential love fuel is low. If we tell someone to rely on you for joy and comfort, we must produce it. Our child is ours. The rest of the world is about their business. You are god in your child's life. When we give birth, we have affirmed our commitment and capability to provide love eternally. Unlike a teenager, a baby cannot up and leave to forage for joy and a purpose to life. "Whatever!" If we refuse to produce joy, let us spare the baby the lingering torture.

We are duty-bound to produce only joy. God says love one another. We must feed our children the security of love. We must immediately set higher standards for ourselves, as regards nurturing our children. It is time high to invest ourselves in the care of our children. It is easy to identify people who have never done a stroke of work with their children. People parents, mothers especially, who are clearly toiling away with their children get asked, the patently ridiculous, "Where do you work?" Now a nanny has a job. A mother is jobless. It is ridiculous a society, so out of touch with the realities of child-rearing, denies us access to abortion.

It is not wrong to choose to die, before nature takes its toll. Neither is it wrong to perform an abortion to spare the unborn the wonderful opportunity to experience the misery of being born unwanted. My greatest issue with abortion bans is this. When a responsible woman decides in the interest of herself and her child, an abortion is necessary, we stall and criminalize her. And yep the slut complex strikes again. We just can't get them out of the equation. Epithets do shape policy. A friend once told me, he is distraught when people call women sluts, except if they are referring to their wives.

Misery is an illegitimate factor in the human existence. Misery is a valid ground to expand access to abortion. The proper motive is what is essential. Life moves on and we reach old age. Always we see, the relatives and the children, who are seeking an out of tending for their families. It is time we see life comprises infinitely more than the puffing of air and cigarettes.

Persons lie comatose in many a hospital. It is a hotly debated subject whether to take them off life support. Keep the focus. The issue is not about allowing the person time, ad infinitum, until death claims them naturally. A reasonable time to allow for the recovery (if practical) of the particular comatose patient should be medically determined. We must exercise patience.Someone would like to have his or her life back. Miracles do happen. We even believe in resurrections.

It is important. We should lose our fascination for maintaining life, in its condition of impotence. We dote on managing impotent and miserable life. As we know there is a historical and present risk of death from pregnancy and childbirth. We risk the lives of perfectly viable mothers daily. Our love for life dictates a ban on childbirth. Every mother's life matters.

Let there be love and let there be the quietness of death. Patients have emerged from comatose. Other patients have never emerged. The issue remains motive. We have decisions to make regarding the death of others. We must accept the responsibility if we have it. It is an immense burden. To all the caretakers, God be blessed. It is only reasonable that we allow the patient a medically reasonable time to recover. This is a guideline. It is only merciful that we allow our family a reasonable time to suffer. As for ending my life? It is mine.

This chapter is hardly about the elderly as it turns out. The regard is for any young or old, who needs a respite from the rigors of living. The disabled among us are love-bound to receive our help, caring, and concern. The need to abort the unborn, scheduled for a date with an unwanted parent, does not contradict our duty to love and care for those already born. The first responsibility of love is to prevent and avoid creating grief. Those who have time, teach their children to say, "Prevention is better than cure", or some variant. If this commitment to prevention finds itself not fully realized, the second duty of love is to treat and hopefully cure the problem.

We shouldn't allow our shortcomings to constitute the basis on which we legislate. It remains valid that we ought not to walk into the life of a two-year-old baby and inform him that his birth was all a big mistake. Now we have arrived to rectify our error. To everything there is a season, a time for every purpose under heaven. This is why I urge on abortion, because born people are not unborn.

I draw again on material from the United States Declaration of Independence. "He has excited domestic insurrections amongst us, and has endeavoured to bring on the inhabitants of our frontiers, the merciless Indian Savages, whose known rule of warfare, is an undistinguished destruction of all ages, sexes and conditions." Let us focus on the "undistinguished destruction of all ages, sexes and conditions." There is hot and cold, rain and shine, night and day, love and hate, good and evil. All boundaries in life are not so clearly defined. Time lives in a warped space. It revels in the blur. Like how do you transition from alive to dead? From conscious to unconscious?

What we know is the human situation evolves from conception to old age. Our human spirit has to calculate the essence of these changes. We have to accept the distinctions pressed upon us. Healthy vs sick. Wanted or unwanted. Loved or abused. Then there is everything else in between. Abortion is about the unavailability of a parent. The child has no mother. She has no mother because her mom does not want to be a mom. If a woman does not want a baby. The baby concurs.

Unborn is the most convenient time to deny another human life. The little person is born, and so it now behooves us to take up the impossible duty and improve on his lot in life. The people who call abortion infanticide are not at all wrong. She is for most of the pregnancy an infant, and she dies. The availability of quality abortion services simply permits the accomplishment of destruction within, instead of without the womb.

A woman has every right to decide if she wishes to be a parent. It is not the woman's right to kill the unborn though. That right belongs to the unborn. Being a parent will always be a personal decision. It is a travesty to need the local court to rule on that. The baby will be born to somebody in particular, who just happens not to be the society. Only a foolish person can make abortion an issue for society to legislate into oblivion.

We know the religious fundamentalists and totalitarian hypocrites are mad. We know they are mad because they presume to tell everybody what books to read, when to have sex, with whom, and sometimes, they tell you how many times. Contrast. The access to abortion does not compel anyone to have abortions. The access to an abortion does not encroach on anyone else's functional ability to bear children. We can still have those lovely religious families. We have to learn to act with speed and decision. Pregnancy is normally nine months long. It is unreasonable to behave as if we have till time immemorial, to secure an abortion. Children are always in immediate need of willing parents. When a baby has cleared the vagina, he has clearly and audibly embarked on a new journey into life. New stage, new negotiations.

It will always be cruel and hypocritical to bear children into deformity and pain, citing the sacred nature of life. When a child is born mentally compromised, should we not crave an improved life for him? An afflicted child remains afflicted, even when we can find him a religious, married, heterosexual couple, who will love him for their own. I accept the society has a legitimate responsibility, to guard the path to death for those already born. The unborn trusts, the society can find the collective courage to leave the path to early death open.

Regarding the elderly being a new target because of abortion. This view can find some validity, if we promote abortions for the convenience of the parents, and not for safeguarding the future of the unborn. The unborn have high expectations. They cannot be disappointed. It pleases us. We rescued a child from an abortion. The job is far from complete. Eternity must find itself invested into the life of the rescued child.

How much like you and me it is to kindle a fire, and then wrangle over the best manner, in which to deal with the fast-spreading, all-consuming blaze. Howl and shriek that an unborn be born to parents, who quarreled over her birth. The children continue to emerge from swollen bellies, ruled by unprepared brains. Still, placards are hoisted. "Stop abortion! Let my people grow, Stop murder." Indeed, we are crazy.

Let us stop murdering the children before we even conceive them. Let my people grow up happy, or let my people not be conceived at all. Stop abortion! Don't be silly. The right to an abortion is a fundamental unborn right. We are desperate to see sexually active women show evidence of their sin. We clothe our concern in rags, self-righteous, selfish rags. The baby, we scream, "Save it." Save it for what. Save it for whom? Save the baby, why? Save the baby for what? Save the baby for whom? In particular. Who are we saving the baby for?

ABORTION NOTES

The Pro-life movement has correctly led us to see it is not a female's right to abort her unborn child. So much more, for a male, to claim abortion as his right. A woman's right to regulate her body and her fertility does not involve the abortion of the unborn. This is fundamental. A woman's right to become a parent is an issue entirely different. This is also fundamental. Pregnancy resets the countenance of all previously enjoyed individual rights. Children need willing parents.

Abortion becomes a female right by proxy. Biologically, pregnancy and childbirth are undisputed woman first, parental responsibilities. Someone must represent the unborn interest. Females are the first responders. Ladies first, this is the unimpeachable biological reality. The jurisdictional food chain flows first, from the keeper of the fetal body. In this chain, the first link is the superior, but not the sole link. There is a good reason even brutes sometimes give up their comforts to a visibly pregnant woman. Interestingly, she might be on the way to an abortion clinic.

It seems selfish and murderously uncaring, for the sexually active to claim the budding human results caused them an inconvenience. Newborn children are the ones being pushed, without their consent, into the vast unknown we call life. I think it only responsible to note our reliability, managing despair, deprivation, and inequality. Nothing dystopian about this, it's just our simple, sugar-coated human history. Oh, how much we need the eternal Pax.

We are not quite discussing tornadoes, drought, hurricanes, volcanoes, earthquakes, floods, pandemics, and other such minor inconveniences of nature. We are discussing the relationships of big people with little people. It can be miserable to survive the fittest. Consider the many things which can go wrong, before children are even born. Just little routine, basic everyday genetic mishaps. Even being born female has been and perhaps still is, one of those congenital defects. It would be patently evil and oppressive for the society, to erect legal walls and procedural minefields, to amputate safe access to contraception and abortion.

To focus abortion, on the parents as murderers is sensational, yes. The murder moniker is one legally identified with globally, and rather easily too. We remain conveniently blind to the punitive plight of the unborn. The young display, in edited and unvarnished reality, their ever available malnutrition of love and affection.

After the British abolished their slave trade in 1807 and the United States in 1808, enterprising planters saw the future of labor. Well-manned breeding farms. Our societies have grown little past that attitude. We perhaps assess children as human numbers. Children are someday to find themselves and occupy their deserved statistical niche, as prince, pauper, or general issue personnel. The planters never cared if their newborn slave knew his father. Okay, sometimes they did. The planters never cared if they later sold mother off, sans enfant. All right, sometimes they did. The planters always cared though that their little slave would be strong, healthy and "normal".

Jesus wept. Those 19th century, Africa processing slave owners turn out to be more merciful than we are. Our hostility towards females is anciently traditional. Our traditional queasiness, with sexual intercourse, makes us very unwilling to care for those whose defiant indulgence openly shows. Unmarried pregnant women have betrayed our happy family. How dare the witch get pregnant and embarrass the family?

An abortion, however, could be even more embarrassing, if not handled in exact professional detail. We are a nation of sexually chaste, responsible persons. We can dislike a woman for playing the whore, getting pregnant, and for putting our secret obsession and pastime on open, swollen display. We dislike a woman for liking sex... just for how it feels. Punishment is only correct for these abominable women. You don't reward these women with an abortion. We let them learn that sexual intercourse has consequences. Babies. Let her handle some responsibility.

Possibly, it may not be mercy or thoughts of compassion for the unborn, which compel us to condemn the abortion procedure, or the contraception procedure. It is more likely, the righteous need to see our compromised neighbor taught a vital life lesson. Responsibility. We call this, "Living up to one's responsibilities." To punish is not our intention. We aim to instill some sexual discipline. Sex is no free ride. That point we must never forget. It does not matter if the married mother used contraception, and it failed. Girls, can't just have fun and get away with it.

Pregnant unwed women should count themselves lucky they are even alive. To punish is honorable, as long as the crime is real, and the punishment is just. Of what crime is the unborn guilty? With whom did the unborn conspire to produce an unwanted, badly timed, poorly planned, ill-conceived pregnancy? This never happens, as we know, life is holy and sacrosanct.

Germany still suffers from its post-Nazi complex. We do too. If we truly hate holocaust, then we could please stop communally capitalizing on greed, and the little skirmishes which leave children bruised, battered, and barely breathing. Like clockwork, crisis is the newborn's assured baby shower. Banning killing does not equal love for life. I don't think anyone wants their newly purchased slave to die before some profit is realised.

After casual examination, it becomes clear, a pregnancy involves mainly a woman and a child. It is clear the baby developing in the woman, develops in stages. It is always human life growing. A fertilized egg is programmed to become a born human being. This human will need caring for. Damn, that unborn human might even be cocky enough to expect a family life. Early abortions, when required, should be socially and legally facilitated, not hindered with word and law games. We know a baby will die. Even when that baby is just a few cells old.

Roe v. Wade did not impose a ban on conception or pregnancy. Roe v. Wade did not declare war on, or debase childbirth, or the raising of families. The Court's decision allows women reasonable time to decide if they wish to be parents. The incubation of human life is first and foremost a female responsibility. The fates of the mother and child physically tie together as soon as pregnancy occurs. The care of the child is overwhelmingly also in the female domain, beginning at breastfeeding. Raising babies is female work. Biology proves this. If women find childcare demeaning, they should have an abortion. The cutting of the umbilical cord signifies the start of a new extended phase of maternal care. Roe v. Wade does not prevent family. This sounds simple and civilized. Simplicity is a good rule of thumb. Simplicity works for the rich and poor alike. For the illiterate and the scholar together. We just can't trump logic.

The near-global obsession, with the sanctity of human life, is a phenomenon, serviced, and conveniently lauded only in the womb. To promote our religious and political agendas, we will willingly dispense with abortion. It only involves a couple of million women and children. If the ghosts of unwanted children somehow mobilized into a powerful political force, demanding abortion, then abortion may suddenly become a reasonable request. Our Legislatures might lend them a quid pro quo ear. I call on spirits because we don't listen to the babies calling 911. The truth is, our legislatures and our finance-driven religious organizations need not lend our abused an ear. A woman gets an abortion when she thinks she is not ready to give a child the quality of life the child deserves. It is the kind, responsible, and motherly action to take. Even a drug-addicted woman understands this.

Children need willing parents. This is sacred. This is the moral standard. This is reality. Religious prejudice and political expediency subjugate blatant human need to vain philosophy. Objective regard for the human situation seems an ancillary consideration in this grand debate.

At the very least, let us embrace honesty, and be direct about our motives, and our concerns governing the abortion issue. Intent we are, in seeing women struggle, with the living burdens of their sin. We pay scant regard to the situation of the child. The innocent child, we say. How do children pay for the indiscretions of the parents? Hopefully not to the third and fourth generations. Men can deposit the sperm, and sometimes the money. No problem here, but the vixen. We carry on our persecution of the female kind. We use our regard for morality and life as our context and pretext. Our grudges against sexually unpalatable women should not manifest in unwanted children.

Pain and misery are about the most hugely produced commodities on earth. Yes, our children continue to feed on hurt and pain. There is a misery surplus in the family trade. A basic premise to establish justice is to ensure the innocent do not suffer for the deeds of the guilty. The innocence of babies. Shouted from prehistoric times. Okay, exaggeration. Today it is justice, we say, to concoct laws condemning innocent children to unwilling parents. The operative term is unwilling. The more frivolous the reason for an abortion, the more urgently we need it facilitated.

We condemn this delicate innocence to the closed arms of parents, who perhaps improperly opened their legs. Our justice is laughable. Were it not for the innocent, we would term our justice ridiculous. Many a score of excellent jokes could not produce laughs so hilarious. Millions of baby lives may be born to taste from nativity limbo. Well, so what? We all know suffering pain is not a sin. Children like their parents to want to have them. As a religious figure well said in modern parlance, "Strain out a fly; swallow a frigging camel."

We care more about protecting the notion of life's sanctity, than in caring for the life. In the United States, the world's abortion activity showpiece. The pro-life movement has conceived of various stratagems to harass and sterilize the potency of Roe v. Wade. There are infinite legal challenges one can concoct to sterilize legal access to abortion. To put it in a military context; guerrilla tactics. Let us discuss a few.

Parental consent is one of the more caring abortion inhibitors. When a very young lady becomes pregnant and seeks an abortion, we need consent, from the other parents, to save that baby from destroying herself. See how long this sentence is? We know it was not her fault; mom and dad are to blame. Abortion always remains the right of the unborn. This is fundamental. It is a natural law. What is any child doing with an eleven or fourteen-year-old mother, fresh out of Barbie Doll University? In more ancient times, and some cultures today, a fourteen-year-old girl would be very much marriageable and thinking about her duties as a wife and mother. Legal and cultural technologies change and sometimes improve.

Today, a Westernized fourteen-year-old is almost too young to pack shelves at the retail store. We want our children to enjoy their childhoods. Not like in these other World places, where there exists child laborers, and children slaves, and child brides. The availability of approved child marriages in the United States of America shows how ingrained our traditions of sexual lunacy are. Abortion as we know is a debate loud, perpetual, and angry. Abortion matters.

Regardless of the age of the parents, particularly that of the mother, abortion remains a basic need for the unborn. Whether teens tell their parents of their pregnancy, abortion remains a required procedure for the benefit of the unborn. As we can see, parents have obvious responsibilities to their minor children. Parents, unless culpable, have decisions to ratify on the behalf of their children, and yes, this also includes abortion.

If the unborn have a right to life, one would expect they have a right to decide when to enjoy that prerogative to life. No parent's wish can overrule the need of the fetus. This is not about might. It is humbly about right. Grandpa or ma should not subordinate the rights of the fetus to his or her wishes. If 14-year-old Luka thinks she needs an abortion, then an abortion she shall get. Go ahead, notify your parents. Just ensure the unborn continue to enjoy unhampered access to the abortionist. The unborn have every right to decide their conception.

We would not step before a moving train, willingly. We are asking an unborn child to do exactly that. Sign up for the gulag. Volunteer for Abu Ghraib prison. Become an indentured servant. Since child parents are so good at the job, why not throw in a few child soldiers?

The fetus has a right to an abortion. As we see from the commonsense of the matter. The fetus's legal jurisdiction lives in an exotic and stoically unborn province. We negotiate it with the intangibles of the law of love, not the shackles of mere laws of conformity.

More legal maneuvers help limit access to abortion. Matters like viability testing and fetal heartbeats. Legislated tests and waiting periods have one major purpose: to frustrate. It adds both time and cost to a once uncomplicated procedure. For abortion, viability is somewhat a non-issue. We find it only prudent to grant the unborn access to abortion. The more viable the unborn, the more demanding our humane commitment. We don't have forever to abort.

The case of the unborn is clear-cut and briskly basic. It takes a few years to grow up, as we all know. Not moot. It is crucial parenthood is a chosen profession, not a social imposition. If the parents are not ready, the baby will wait until they are. Viability testing is a non-issue in this trade of death. Viability testing is relevant only to those who enjoy playing practical jokes in life or death situations. Abortion is an issue of death, par excellence... and so is life. Family, not giving birth, sanctifies unborn life.

There is yet another instrument used to help engineer a decline in the number of abortions. The withdrawal of government and state funding for facilities, or organizations providing abortion. The intent is to say, "The buck stops here and so does abortion." The implications of this tactic are weighty and far-reaching. In conclusion. It is the government's money.

Every society benefits from children who receive proper care. Pregnancies should not be encouraged to the birth stage, with the coerced cooperation of the hostage future parents. Whatever happened to family? This manner of harassment to the rights of the unborn is intolerable.

Finally, we arrive at informed consent. This informed consent is the propaganda blade of this many-pronged, anti-abortion fork. The concept operates by demanding women receive education, showing the horror abortion wreaks on the poor unborn, and the female reproductive "facilities". This is a marvelous idea, but not to discourage women from aborting the pregnancy they already have. We should also show images of recently abused and despondent children. We should show also the corpses of the emaciated two-year-olds.

We should show the dirt poor abused ladies. We should show the borderline, clinically sane women trying to juggle a paycheck and childcare. Just one or two should do. We should show the battered bodies of children tortured, emotionally and otherwise, by demented care. We should ensure delivery rooms have ever looping audio of the shrieks and screams of our unwanted offspring. We should show what can go wrong after the ultrasound.

We can show the moms who just don't want a baby, but who have had one, anyway. As pointed out earlier. We strip no intellectual property from the unborn. Abortion can be a very nasty business. Life for sure is always a very nasty business. You better have good help and good luck navigating.

Pretend, children do not live life abused. Imagine life is wonderful. Persuade yourself. A child's greatest known trauma is to be force-fed broccoli. Frank and graphic representation of the horror of some abortions may help reduce future abortions.

Come to think of it, frank and graphic representations of child abuse might help with contraception use too.

When a woman plans to have a baby, should the hospital bottle feed her material, showing the perils of pregnancy, motherhood, marriage, and the many evils, which may likely befall the child? There is no easy end to the terrible, heart-wrenching possibilities, facing children who are born. Fewer unwanted pregnancies should help reduce the abortion figures. Now that's what we all want. Isn't it? Human life begins at contraception.

Does the father of the child have to make himself available for informing? Let the gentleman join the women during the procedure, or pay a fine. We are present to help with conception, why should we not be present at the death. We are comfortable enough with each other to have sex and conceive a life. It is no great deal to supervise our kill together. If we were having a simple graduation ceremony, we would shoot a camera full of memories. Weddings bask in a perpetual glow of flashbulbs. Let us also remember the day we regrettably or callously killed, or murdered the tiny tot. Vote informed consent, if it makes the legislatures feel better.

People want abortions because they want to end a pregnancy. Perhaps, someone might not want her child to be born into oppression. Perhaps, someone might not want to be pregnant for the current father. Perhaps, someone wants to prepare for drug rehab, for example. Perhaps someone wants to go to school. Perhaps someone wants a work promotion. You know, all the little mundane stuff, which turns out to be devastatingly and intimately relevant to the unborn. From the first pregnant moment, we know abortion kills the baby to be. No room for semantics there. What do we want to inform about? There is a very proper choice when parenthood is unwanted. Abortion.

Have you ever met a single mom, and her smiling child, or children? The love, the pride, and the joy of her life. It makes you smile too. So why not this argument? If the lady had used contraception that child would never have been born. If she did not have the sweet baby, out of wedlock, the child would never have been born. If she did not have that second baby, while she struggled to care for the first, the baby would never have been born.

This is also why we must legally guarantee, and enforce equal work, equal pay. God says, "By the sweat of your brow shall you eat bread." How does the mother pay for the care of the child? Being a single mother is hard enough. Being a broke single mother is harder still. As you would expect, we especially don't recommend single parenthood. Life begins at contraception.

Abortion remains critically an issue of unborn care and concern. Abortion is not a communicable disease.

Your wife does not catch abortion, because my wife just had an abortion. Abortion is no coronavirus.

None of us are morally qualified to deny an unborn child an abortion.

It is easy to understand. Children should be born to people who want to be parents. To be a parent, this is a tall order. There is nothing intelligent about forced parenthood. Forcing parenting is child abuse. Please note. Family is not born, just because we get pregnant and make babies. God invented family. It should be easy for religious people to understand family planning. Life, out of respect for itself, begins at contraception.

BE OF GOOD CHEER.

L et this debate consider a cease and let joy multiply. Joy, because we went to bed with responsibility embraced. Joy, for Family walked by, and we sang it our praises. Disperse joy wide and far. Receive the joy. It is available to be tasted. The immorality has ceased. The disciplined rejoice in their purity. The chaste are eager to spread both legs and joy, in the family's holy context.

Multiply joy, for selfish copulations no longer stand poised. None to blight and poison that tender population. Joy is multiplied, for no births of thoughtless design are added. Joy, we add joy. The illegitimacy of shame, and its attendant pain has been subtracted. Joy be multiplied. No more are the children born to parents divided.

Our joy is multiplied. The children are happy to wake. The tots are secretly pleased to be disturbed. The babes hope for rousing. The young ones listen for an excuse to wipe the sleep from shiny eyes. The little ones desire to wake. So they may gaze with joy at that happy pair who brought them here.

Life grows large with pleasure, pain shrinks to insignificant measure, when our children's' lives with love we insure. A pregnancy, a teeny weeny one just yet, appeared sometime after a conjugal fete. Liquid joy from eyes flowed, and hands were tightly clasped, not in grief, and not in fear. Her mouth grappled at first with speech, but still the obvious she managed to share, "Sweetie, I think we have that other pregnancy."

Love dripped from your honey lips, I regarded it. Passion throbbed from beneath your chest. There I placed my ear. Love beat a secret code in your heart, and it echoed in mine. Comfort whispered from your gentle hand, so there I placed my ear.

The toes curled with pleasure, and then tapped to me, the encouragement of your love. To your feet, I placed my ear. Have you ever wondered, my baby dear, why I always placed my ear? It is because, whatever you were saying, I wanted to hear.

The End.

ACKNOWLEDGEMENT

Scripture quotations from or based on King James Version.

BOOKS BY THIS AUTHOR

Christopher Colombus The Legal Voyage

Quasi, Historical Stage play.

Herod & The Birth Of Christmas

Quasi, Historical Stage Play.

Star Spangled Banner Unstrangled

Short Prose.

www.ingramcontent.com/pod-product-compliance
Lightning Source LLC
Chambersburg PA
CBHW031103250726

48655CB00004B/1565